Making a New Countryside

Astri Andresen
Josep L. Barona
Steven Cherry
(eds.)

Making a New Countryside

Health Policies and Practices in European History ca. 1860–1950

PETER LANG
Frankfurt am Main · Berlin · Bern · Bruxelles · New York · Oxford · Wien

Bibliographic Information published by the Deutsche Nationalbibliothek
The Deutsche Nationalbibliothek lists this publication in the Deutsche Nationalbibliografie; detailed bibliographic data is available in the internet at http://dnb.d-nb.de.

Cover design:
Olaf Glöckler, Atelier Platen, Friedberg

This book has been supported
by the Spanish Ministry of Science and Technology
(MICIN HAR 2008-0012-E)

ISBN 978-3-631-59653-1

www.peterlang.de

CONTENTS

CONTRIBUTORS

Astri Andresen is Professor in History at Department of Archaeology, History, Cultural studies and Religion at the University of Bergen. She is researching Sámi history, history of children and childhood and of health and medicine.

María-José Báguena is Senior Lecturer in History of Science at the Instituto de Historia de la Medicina y de la Ciencia López Piñero (Universitat de València-CSIC). Her research focuses on the history of infectious diseases, public health and Valencian medicine. She is a member of the Board of the Spanish Society for the History of Medicine and secretary of *Cronos.*

Rosa Ballester is Professor of the History of Medicine at the University Miguel Hernández in Alicante. Her research has focused on European paediatrics in a hisorical perspective, as well as public health issues on malaria and poliomyelitis.

Josep L. Barona is Professor of History of Science and Head of the Department of History of Science and Documentation, Universitat de València. His research topics include international health, rural health and nutrition in Europe and Spanish scientific exile. Among his last publications are *Health and Medicine in Rural Europe*, co-edited with Steven Cherry and *La Salud y el Estado. La administración española y el movimiento sanitario internacional* (2008) in collaboration with Josep Bernabeu.

Josep Bernabeu-Mestre is Professor of the History of Science at the University of Alicante. His principal field of research is the history of the public health, particularly in relation to nutrition, mother and child health care and historical epidemiology in contemporary Spain.

Steven Cherry is Reader in the History of Medicine, the School of History, University of East Anglia, Norwich. His published research includes the history of mental health care; medical services and the hospitals.

Angela Cremades Monerris is a nurse and PhD student in the Program of Public Health of the University of Alicante.

Josep X. Esplugues is Assistant Professor of the History of Science at the University of Alicante. His principal field of research is the historical epidemiology and the history of nutrition.

María E. Galiana is Community Nursing Professor at the University of Alicante (Spain). Her principal fields of research are the history of rural and environmental health and nursing and child health care in the contemporary Spain.

Tore Grønlie is Professor of Modern History at the University of Bergen. He has published books and articles on the history of health, medicine and welfare, governance, public administration, public enterprise and local self-government in 20th century Scandinavia.

Joaquim Guillem-Llobat is a postdoctoral research associate at the Department of History of Science and Documentation, Universitat de València. His research focuses on European food history in the late nineteenth and early twentieth century.

Paola M. Melis is a researcher paticipating in a multidisciplinary research project on 'genetic isolates' in the Ogliastra region, Sardinia, carried out by the Institute of Population Genetics in Sassari and the Italian National Research Council.

Lucia Pozzi is Professor of Demography in the Faculty of Economics, University of Sassari and president of the Italian Society of Historical Demography. Among her last publications are *La lotta per la vita* (2000) and co-edited with M. Breschi: *Salute, malattia e sopravvivenza in Italia `800 e `900* (2007) and *The determinants of infant and child mortality in past European Populations* (2004).

Esteban Rodriguez-Ocaña is Professor of History of Science at the University of Granada. He is former President of the European Association for the History of Medicine (2001-03), and as member of the Interwar Health Network he has co-edited, with Patrick Zylberman, the dossier 'Improving Public Health Amidst Crises: The Interwar Years in Europe' in *Dynamis*, 2008; 28. Currently he serves in the editorial boards of Asclepio (Madrid), História-Ciências-Saúde (Rio de Janeiro), and Medical Humanities (London).

Catherine Rollet is Professor at the University of Versailles Saint-Quentin-en-Yvelines and member of the CNRS (Printemps). She is a specialist in the history of children and demography. Among her last publications are: *Les enfants au XIXe siècle* (2001), *La population du monde, 6 milliards et demi, et demain?* (2006) and *Les carnets de santé des enfants* (2008).

María-Isabel Porras-Gallo is Senior Lecturer in History of Science in the Departamento de Ciencias Médicas at the Universidad de Castilla la Mancha. Her main research fields are the history of diseases, the history of physical disabilities and social protection.

Teemu Ryymin is Senior Researcher at Stein Rokkan Centre for Social Studies, Unifob, Bergen. His research topics include history of health and medicine in 19th and 20th century Norway, particularly tuberculosis prevention, history of medical institutions and rural health. He has worked extensively on the history of ethnic minorities in Northern Scandinavia.

INTRODUCTION: 'RURAL HEALTH' AS A EUROPEAN HISTORICAL ISSUE

Astri Andresen, Josep L. Barona and Steven Cherry

In the nineteenth and early twentieth centuries the majority of Europeans lived in rural societies; societies that in a multitude of ways differed from cities and towns. Some of the differences were conceived as affecting issues pertaining to health, while others no doubt had a direct impact. For example, the nineteenth-century favourable differential in rural infant mortality rates is well known and documented, as are, conversely, the perceived advantages for urban populations in accessing available health services.[1]

Albeit with an emphasis on Spain, this volume aims at establishing new knowledge about how and why 'the rural' emerged as a medico-political problem, and how the problem was tackled in states positioned in different parts of Europe: England and Scotland to the west, France, Italy and Spain more to the south, and Norway to the north – and also in different time periods. Such knowledge, obviously, offers a path to understanding the history of health differences and contrasts in the range of service provision for various groups of the population, and we believe it also increases the understanding of the cultural construction of Europe from the late nineteenth century until World War Two. In particular, the volume demonstrates that the position of 'the rural' in European cultures was ambiguous: on the one hand representing the good, the clean and the unspoilt – morally as well as physically – yet also being perceived as backwards, uncivilised and on the absolute margins of 'the modern'. With this ambiguity in mind, the book addresses a vital issue in medical history: how have medical science and medical practitioners contributed to the making of concepts describing places, spaces and populations? To what extent were these contributions important in changing people's lives?

The editors and many contributors to this volume have been involved in common research on the history of rural health since 2003, when Steven Cherry outlined an emerging historiographical approach and suggested collaborative research from an international perspective. Consequently, several colloquia, conference panels and monographs have been published by members of an informal European network on the history of rural health in Europe since c. 1800, promoted by history of medicine and health groups at our respective Universi-

1 E.g. Hubbard, W. et al. *Historical Studies in Mortality Decline*, Oslo, Det Norske Videnskaps-Akademi, 2002.

ties.[2] In October 2008 the Valencia Colloquium on *Health and the Rural in Europe (1860-1970), Organisations, Practices and Campaigns* took place around four themes: 'Health and Living Conditions', 'Health Care Organisations and Practices', 'Child Health Policy' and 'Epidemiology and Sanitary Campaigns'. Versions of papers read at the meeting are included in this volume but, since all the contributions in one way or other dealt with the political history of health or policy considerations of some kind, the original thematic sub-division has not been retained.

The authors discuss rural health policies – or in some case their absence – at local, regional or national levels; covering sanitary and social campaigns, legislation and regulation, and the establishment and functioning of certain health services. Some authors also investigate the relationship between international and national or local agencies but, in particular, all consider which reforms were deemed necessary and by whom, and why, if and how these were implemented. Many issues were common to all or most Western countries; for example mother and child health care, the fight against diseases like poliomyelitis, and food control. Others, like trachoma and malaria, were specific to certain areas. But as a whole, rural districts and rural health are considered a complex field of social, cultural and scientific interaction in which a wide range of agents, interests, values and ideologies intervened. Of course, many of the 'rural' measures discussed or implemented were associated with programmes to improve urban health, confirming previous findings that it was common for urban-based initiatives to be exported to the countryside, albeit sometimes in modified form. The entire public health field offers an example of such export, as do school medical services and school meals.

The hygienisation of the countryside implied almost everywhere three levels of intervention: political, social and technical, all investigated in chapters below. Interventions were increasingly based upon laboratory research and utilised vital statistics, involving various health care facilities and sanitary campaigns. Thus, increasingly, science played a vital role. Agencies and the levels of action might vary from local communities on the one hand to those involving international

---

2 In autumn 2003 a Colloquium on 'Rural Health and Medical Care' took place at the University of East Anglia co-ordinated by Steven Cherry and Josep L. Barona and a second meeting took place in Valencia in November 2004 including the history of health and medicine group of the University of Bergen. Since then, an informal international network involving the Universities of Bergen, East Anglia and Valencia has promoted publications, colloquia and session panels in international conferences on rural health, such as the European Association for the History of Medicine and Health (Paris, 2005 and London, 2007); and the Bergen workshop on the History of Health and Medicine (2006). Authors have contributed to a special issue of the *International Journal of Local and Regional Studies* (2006).

organisations on the other, acting alongside local and national administrations and with the involvement of voluntary and philanthropic organisations.

The first chapter in this book, written by Paola Melis and Lucia Pozzi, investigates health conditions and social inequality in Sardinia, seeking to document the health status of populations not only rural, but also poor, and making explicit the connection between health, livelihood and policies, highlighting trachoma and dietary deficiencies. It offers a substantial contribution to knowledge of living conditions and ill-health in what might be regarded as a part of the Italian periphery, showing on the one hand how poverty and bad communications had detrimental effects upon health, and on the other hand the impotence of political and medical authorities in changing the situation.

In the next two chapters, Steven Cherry and Josep Barona deal with rural health policies in general over most of the time period under investigation. Cherry's chapter adopts a comparative approach, taking a rural area and one undergoing industrialisation but focusing upon a neglected actor, the rural medical officer of health in England and Scotland, and demonstrating the value of appreciating the local context when considering policy implementation. Barona's chapter discusses the origins of Spain's liberal reforms and the configuration of a sanitary movement to cope with poverty, disease and bad living conditions in urban and rural areas during the last years of the nineteenth century. He pays special attention to health care reforms in rural districts during the Spanish Republican period (1931-1939), when rural health became a major part of the 'civilising programme' of Spanish society in the context of the post-1929 international crisis.

The following chapters discuss particular aspects of rural health policies over shorter periods of time. Esteban Rodrigues-Ocaña investigates the role of the *Inspección de Sanidad del Campo*, the Rural Health Office in Spain, active between 1910 and 1918 and focused on rural areas, but outside the remit of the National Health Department. It was associated with early proposals for health surveillance, which included both diseases and environmental and social conditions, but represents an example of an ambitious scheme that failed, reflecting the wider political and administrative situation.

The prevention and eradication of two particular diseases, trachoma and polio, are investigated in chapters by Maria Eugenia Galiana, Angela Cremades and Josep Bernabeu-Mestre and by Maria José Báguena, Maria Isabel Porras and Rosa Ballester respectively. Both diseases represented huge health problems (trachoma, cf. also Melis and Pozzi) and are examined from a rural-urban and, in the case of polio, from a national perspective. It is indicated that the fight against trachoma was not eagerly supported by the populations in question – obviously an issue for further research – and the authors conclude that for this reason, active detection of cases was needed, as was work to modify risk factors. Baguena, Porras and Ballester offer a study of Spanish polio history that investigates which medical and political meaning was given to the environment and also highlights the potential political usefulness for the Francoist regime of a disease that was understood as a 'disease of civilisation'.

Ximo Guillem's chapter is concerned with changes in the food chain. Comparing food safety in rural and urban contexts, he suggests that, on this issue, rural communities had some advantages over urban ones. It was urban societies that experienced the most dramatic changes in the food chain and, thus, were also most at risk of food fraud. However, they were also the first to introduce in particular chemical analysis to detect such frauds – while the countryside more or less relied for a long period upon traditional organoleptic methods.

In her chapter Catherine Rollet investigates a century of child health policies in France, in particular the farming out of children from the major cities to the countryside, thus demonstrating shifting evaluations of 'the rural' and the implications of these changes. Her paper shows how, between the two world wars, the previously under-equipped countryside began to benefit from a programme of economic and medico-social development, vastly improving health and living conditions. The link between Rollet's contribution and the chapter by Astri Andresen and Teemu Ryymin is that both analyse policies to create greater equality in public health and access to health services between rural and urban municipalities and different regions. Andresen and Ryymin focus upon the expansion of a system of medical officers of health and the establishment of health institutions in the countryside, in particular tuberculosis homes and cottage hospitals.[3] Local agency was particularly important to the establishment of such hospitals, and also in defending the entire system of public health and health care during the interwar crisis. In the final chapter, Tore Grønlie outlines the urban-rural distribution of general hospital services in Norway in the decades 1920 to 1950. His focus is not upon political aims, but upon how the general hospital needs of rural or peripheral populations were actually met, relative to those of urban dwellers. Somewhat unexpectedly, he finds that access to hospitals was not defined as a particular problem for rural patients, but the costs were, as was the degree of specialisation. This was low, and Grønlie indicates that a decentralised structure with good access came at a price; the low degree of specialisation and also a low degree of formal hierarchies between the various institutions.

---

3 For rural hospitals and medical officers of health, see also Cherry, S. 'General practitioners, Hospitals and Medical Services in Rural England: the East Anglia Region c. 1800-1948', in Barona, J.L. and Cherry, S. (eds.) *Health and Medicine in Rural Europe 1860-1945*, Valencia, PUV/SEC, 2005.

Differences and commonalities

When looking at health policies, sickness and health and the living conditions of rural populations in areas as distant as Ogliastra in Sardinia, Norfolk in England, Valenica and Castilia in Spain or Finnmark in Norway in the late nineteenth and early twentieth centuries, we face plural realities and no one factor explains their differences. We have discussed issues concerning differences and commonalities in earlier publications,[4] but let us here point to some factors of particular importance regarding the chapters in this book. Most obviously, the various locations differ with respect to geography, topography and climate; factors that are highly relevant with regard both to prevailing diseases and the distribution of health services. Second, they differ with respect to demography, economy and social structures; vital in regard to what a country could do – or was prepared to do – in safeguarding the health of its inhabitants. It should of course also be emphasised that differences at national level might be huge, both between different classes and between regions, the latter demonstrated in the chapters by Andresen and Ryymin and Grønlie.

Third and obviously, countries had different modes of government and experienced varying levels of stability or upheaval in the period.[5] By 1936 Mussolini had consolidated in fascist Italy and Spain began to be wreaked by the Civil War, whereas in Norway the labour party had its first anniversary in office, supported by the agrarian party. Except for Norway and Spain, all countries were involved in World War One and, barring Spain, also in World War Two – wars that in numerous ways changed Europe and European policies. Particularly important in regard to health was first, the interwar economic crisis and, second, that social help was gradually replaced by state welfare schemes in Britain and Norway; substituting concepts of entitlement as of right for earlier notions of assistance and charity. The two Norwegian chapters here cover the transition from the social help state to the welfare state, indicating also the role of rural agencies and the position of rural societies in this process.

Finally, and related to these developments, it is important to emphasise the extent to which the social and political position of rural populations in Europe

---

4 Cf. Cherry, S. 'Medicine and Rural Health Care in 19th Century Europe' and Andresen, A. 'Perspectives on the Interaction of Medicine and Rural Cultures: Spain, Norway and European Russia 1860s-1910s', both in Barona and Cherry (eds.) *Health and Medicine in Rural Europe.* When it comes to demographic differences between various European regions, a considerable amount of research has been published, but for the impact of different economic and demographic regimes upon social difference and how people handled their lives, see Henderson, J. and Wall, R. (eds) *Poor Women and Children in the European past,* London, Routledge, 1994.

5 See also, for example, the Introductory Survey in Borowy, I. and Gruner, W.D. (eds.) *Facing illness in troubled times: health in Europe in the interwar years 1918-1939,* Frankfurt am Main and New York, Peter Lang, 2005.

also varied. The extreme marginalisation economically and politically of some rural societies and their inhabitants that Italian and Spanish contributors point out might be contrasted with Norway, where free farmers were considered as the backbone of that country's cultural nationalism and representatives elected by the (male) farmers actually dominated its Parliament from 1814 well into the interwar period. One should note, though, that in Norway, there was an almost continuous battle over cultural values but, even so, the extent to which 'civilisation' was a common theme everywhere is striking. The 'civilisation process' is evident in several chapters in this volume, as previous research has demonstrated it was in Norway until the early years of the twentieth century.[6]

Despite differences, the images of rural populations and of rural health problems produced in different times and places call for comparative reflections over 'the rural', not least because they affected the respective solutions prescribed by medical practitioners and local, national and international authorities. To civilise, cultivate or modernise rural populations was a general project from the middle or late nineteenth century and, in varying but also modified forms, throughout the interwar period in all the countries in question. Without necessarily being produced at the same time, descriptions of, for example, rural hygiene varied more in scale than in content. We do not suggest the imagery reflected rural life and rural health as contrasted to urban life and urban health but, rather, that rural populations were spoken of in a similar language in different parts of Europe because certain specific ideas had been circulated, if not created, internationally. Thus we believe that, at the time when biology became increasingly important in explaining differences between populations or 'races', the purported different levels of civilisation received such attention because they might account for variations within populations otherwise defined as unitary, for example as Spanish or Norwegian. This takes us on to the broader conceptualisation of the place of 'the rural' in promoting health or spreading diseases – and the profound shifts it underwent in the nineteenth and first part of the twentieth century.

From idealisation to condemnation

The idealisation of Nature has deep roots in western tradition, playing an important part in the conceptions of health and disease in Hellenic natural philosophy and Hippocratic medicine. The conceptualisation of health as balanced harmony linked to environmental conditions was a central point in the Hippocratic treatise on 'Airs, waters and places', making understandable the healing power of Nature. Under this health ideology, sun, water, fresh air, heat, cold, diet and exercise were the main healing factors to prevent and cure disease. This tradition

6 Andresen, A. and Ryymin, T. 'Towards Equality? Rural Health and Health Acts in Norway, 1860-1912', in Barona and Cherry (eds.) *Health and Medicine in Rural Europe*.

contributed to building a positive image of rural life associated with the healing power of Nature.

The construction of the 'noble savage' from the seventeenth century and the Romantic idealisation of Nature in early contemporary times also emphasised nature as a positive factor, indeed part of the making of the 'healthy' and 'unspoilt' rural. A series of social and medical initiatives in the second half of the nineteenth century; school camps, sea sanatoria, spa institutions, open air schools and sport associations, convalescent homes, excursion clubs, sanatoria for tuberculosis patients and institutions for polio victims, shared this common idea of the healing influence of nature and a positive image of the countryside as a source of health. Thus, the clean, healthy rural is an old construction that experienced a new boost in the late nineteenth century, as seen in several of the contributions to this book, and not least so because the countryside was contrasted with urban environments marked by industrialisation and a disordered rise of the population.

But at the same time, changing perceptions of the rural were resulting in its depiction as a dirty, backward space (cf. in particular Barona's and Cherry's chapters). Several factors influenced the making of this different image: notably new values associated with modernity, cosmopolitanism and progress; the differences in living conditions between urban and rural societies and a lack of modern facilities that made life easier in urban than in rural surroundings. Critical to this shift in perception were scientific theories drawn from bacteriology, alongside more contestable views derived from the several versions of Social Darwinism and theories of degeneration. Together, they contributed to the perception of the rural as a contaminated and underdeveloped space that threatened the strength of the respective countries, although many campaigns against disease in rural populations were based not upon new medical reasoning but derived from older views that 'contagion' essentially reflected an insufficiently civilised way of life. To various degrees in different countries medical topographies, reports from rural and colonial medicine, as well as social reports and health conferences, underpinned this approach.[7]

Experimental scientific knowledge and vital statistics increasingly contributed to a change of perception. Laboratory medicine, with its hygienists, health officers and experimental technicians, played a vital role in providing a new expertise. Scientific theories were in some countries justified by vital statistics, with epidemiological data and anthropometrical records pointing to rural inferiority in life standards and health conditions, as some of the chapters in this volume point out. An image of a sick, polluted and backward rural thus appeared, competing with the earlier healthy rural. To some extent this perception was also sharply contrasted with that of more 'civilised' urban societies. Some ambiva-

7 Barona and Cherry (eds.) *Health and Medicine in Rural Europe.*

lence remained regarding both rural and urban societies; for example, in practice views of the urban and rural working classes did not necessarily differ that much. What was different, though, was that urban space seemed to be under more rigorous inspection than rural space, with public health being more systematically pursued.

In most European states central administrations translated new concepts and urban values into political measures to promote health. As a political programme, rural health may be analysed as a scientific and a social endeavour, but also as a civilising process, defined by Norbert Elias as one in which external social constraints proscribing behaviours gradually became internalised; accompanied by feelings of shame directed inward and of repugnance directed towards the others.[8] He suggested that, in modern Western culture, behaviour associated with the body came to be strictly regulated. External prohibitions became internalised, while violations occasioned not only social punishment but also shame in the transgressor and disgust in others. From this perspective, the late nineteenth and early twentieth centuries appear as a crucial stage in a process to change the countryside; making it more similar to cities and towns. In this respect, sanitary campaigns could thus also be considered an element in the battle to move the peasantry forward along the cultural path from backwardness to civilisation.[9]

Health and living conditions provided physicians and politicians with some key arguments why hygienisation via civilisation was of utmost importance. Health, along with education, became a principal field for social action, with the growing assumption that only civilised people could attain the rights and benefits of citizenship and membership in the community of healthy, working human beings: an issue of particular importance as democratically elected governments were introduced.

Health policies, medical science and bacteriology in particular served also in the colonial enterprise, as they did in urban slums and poor rural societies. The French case is in this respect telling: seven Pasteur Institutes were set up in the colonies between 1891 and 1914 and a network of national and provincial institutes of health was established all over Europe during these years. Urban and

8 Elias, N. *Über den Prozeß der Zivilisation. Soziogenetische und psychogenetische Untersuchungen. Erster Band. Wandlungen des Verhaltens in den weltlichen Oberschichten des Abendlandes* and *Zweiter Band. Wandlungen der Gesellschaft. Entwurf einer Theorie der Zivilisation*, Basel, Verlag Haus zum Falken, 1939 (Published in English as *The Civilizing Process, Vol.I. The History of Manners*, Oxford, Blackwell, 1969, and *The Civilizing Process, Vol.II. State Formation and Civilization*, Oxford, Blackwell, 1982); Barnes, D.S. *The Great Stink of Paris and the Nineteenth-Century Struggle against Filth and Germ*, Baltimore, The Johns Hopkins University Press, 2006.

9 Barnes, *The Great Stink of Paris*; Labisch, A. *Homo Hygienicus. Gesundheit und Medizin in der Neuzeit*, Frankfurt, Campus, 1992.

rural health officers, local and national administrators, took part in the same 'civilising mission'. Disinfection programmes, vaccination campaigns, bacteriological laboratories and rural health centres all show how public health was enjoined with scientific progress as a means of conquering poverty and dirtiness. By the early twentieth century, health programmes in all the countries under discussion had become part of national policies.

The chapters of this book certainly serve to demonstrate European variation and the multiple meanings of sickness, health and political agency. But they also suggest commonalities, not only in the use of an imagery of civilisation but in that health policies were increasingly seen as emblematic for the level of 'modernisation' and as a yardstick by which to compare not only rural and urban communities, but different states. The Finnish historian Pauli Kettunen has argued that both the nation state and modernisation 'gained ever more ground as universal principles in the course of the nineteenth century' and came to 'provide the transnational preconditions and contexts for international comparisons'.[10] The way that Spain in the period 1931-33 turned to international organisations for scientific and systems advice is a prime example; as is the way in which poliomyelitis was handled as a political issue under the Franco-regime. Thus, even if this volume does not set out systematically to compare health, living conditions and health policies, it is important to emphasise that comparisons were used as a political tool, with rural health receiving increased attention and international competition recognised as one important feature involved.

Science and government

What then, were the main rural problems addressed by medicine in the late nineteenth and early twentieth century? Medical topographies generally described rural housing as falling below the most elementary standards of civilised and hygienic living. Besides, peasants were often depicted as mistrusting physical and moral progress and rejecting changes in their habits; just the opposite of town- or city-dwellers, 'where people improve their situation by taking intelligent care of themselves'.[11] Around 1880, when the bacteriological doctrine of contagion became widely accepted, a key factor was added to negative perceptions of both the urban poor and rural populations: the attempt to link dirtiness and non-hygienic lifestyles with disease by means of a specific germ. By introducing the identifiability of disease-specific germs through laboratory techniques, bacteriology opened a new front in the battle against infectious diseases. However, the spread of the bacteriological thinking did not necessarily contra-

---

10 Kettunen, P. 'The power of international comparison', in Christiansen, N.F., Petersen, K. Edling, N. and Haave, P. (eds.) *The Nordic Model of Welfare A Historical Reappraisal*, Copenhagen, Museum Tusculanum Press, 2006.

11 Barnes, *The Great Stink*.

dict previous conceptions since laboratory medicine did not oppose but often complemented the moralistic dimension of dirtiness and transgression.

David Barnes suggested that the late nineteenth-century imperative of cleanliness, born as a social code, was reinforced by experimental science so that public health concerns were strengthened and followed a more bacteriological orientation.[12] The mutual influence of medical knowledge and moral principles played a central role in the making of this sanitary-bacteriological synthesis. Some authors have connected dirtiness and the banishment of excrement associated with disease transmission and microbes with disgust among the respectable bourgeoisie.[13] The recognition of germs as specific, identifiable causes added a qualitative difference to the traditional link between dirtiness and disease. When pathogenic microbes were found in excrements, bodily excretions, drinking water, infected food, and other substances they became the main target of hygienists' action. Rural districts were now depicted as the most unhygienic spaces endowed with a number of negative attributes: overcrowded houses, the co-mingling of humans with animals, manure heaps and uncontrolled defecation. To this was often added ignorance, defective and unbalanced diet and high alcohol consumption: in short, peasant life became the archetype of unhealthy living and backwardness.

In particular the intimacy of humans and animals threatened with contamination by infectious microbes was emphasised. In the hot season, flies and other insects left germs on food and water and further polluted the air. Whereas animals represented a source of wealth for the peasantry they were now also depicted as a threat, their separation or even elimination being indispensable to avoid contagious diseases. This hygienic ideology was absolutely opposite to a rural way of life and mentality that valued animals and their manure as essential to agricultural prosperity. With microbes directly verifiable through experimental methods, manure achieved pathogenic consistency, recognised as a health hazard as well as an agricultural resource. Yet this social ideology emerging around cleanliness also influenced peasant life and values, although it to some extent was contradictory with traditional rural life: it is difficult to assess the attitudes of peasants as a whole but some had rising expectations regarding cleanliness and these were not exclusively imposed by authoritarian hygienists, medical officers, the urban bourgeoisie, health administrators and politicians.[14]

---

12 Barnes, *The Great Stink*, 198-205.

13 Barona and Cherry (eds), *Health and Medicine*; Barnes, *The Great Stink*, 211-217; Worboys, M. *Spreading Germs: disease theories and medical practice in Britain 1865-1900*, Cambridge, Cambridge University Press, 2002.

14 How hygienisation campaigns were received is not further investigated in this volume although it constitutes an important aspect for comparison among countries, cultures and civil attitudes regarding authority and expertise in contemporary Europe. A starting point is

Considering the serious social and economic dimension of infectious diseases in the early twentieth century, the hygienist universe built a strong ideology against dirtiness and filth as main causes, based on the consistency contributed by bacteriology. This feature is critical to understanding the enduring strength of the sanitary-bacteriological synthesis, with the two elements of filth/contamination and germs as inseparable. Nevertheless, Barnes notes that:

> 'the training of the senses that made the crusade against filth possible must be attributed principally to long-term cultural change, although medical science certainly added to its momentum by finding new reasons to denounce transgressions against the hygienic code of separation and containment. But there were still other historical forces that shaped the cleanliness impulse in late nineteenth-century public health. Chief among them was the social renegotiation that attempted to integrate the peasantry fully into a modern national identity.'[15]

This is important in understanding the different developments in European countries. In some, the peasantry definitely represented 'the other' but elsewhere it might be regarded as uncivilised yet at the same time constituting the mainstay of national identity. This difference might explain some of the varied approaches to rural health evident in this volume.

Yet some standards in the creation of sanitary and hygienic societies had been set long ago. The *Déclaration des Droits de l'Homme* was the starting point for the establishment of a *Comité de Salubrité* (1790) in France, devoted to vigilance concerning popular health and the operation of sanitary institutions. One member, Louis René Villermé, published several reports on the social dimension of disease at the *Académie de Medicine* and *Académie des Sciences Morales et Politiques*. He explored hygienic conditions in prisons and in different Paris districts, identifying diseases affecting local poor populations and the features of moral and physical degradation in the working classes in reports which thus linked poverty, exclusion, living conditions, mortality and disease.[16]

Edwin Chadwick and the British *Sanitary Movement*, inspired by Bentham's Utilitarianism, also emphasised the importance of social factors in the distribution of disease among population groups. William Farr published his *Vital Statistics* (1839) in McCulloch's remarkable work *A Statistical Account of the British Empire* (1842), which raised awareness of the lower classes' sanitary

---

Baldwin, P. *Contagion and the State in Europe 1830-1930*, Cambridge, Cambridge University Press, 1999.

15 Barnes, *The Great Stink*, 211.

16 Rosen, G. 'Mercantilism and Health Policy in Eighteenth Century French Thought', *Medical History, 3,* (1959), 259-277. See also La Berge, A. F. 'The early 19th century French Public Health Movement', *Bulletin of the History of Medicine* 58, (1984), 3, 363-379.

problems. Health statistics were a major contribution, since epidemiological indicators and surveys on workers' health conditions provided new concepts such as *life expectancy* and conceptualised hygienic impairment. [17]

In Germany, *cameralism* reshaped former *medizinische Polizei* programmes and in the mid nineteenth century several *Länder* started a process of sanitary reform focused upon state organisation of public health services. A national Ministry of Health was created as early as 1871, later followed by the establishment of state health insurance (*Krankenkassen)* as one expression of Bismarckian measures to offset the growing influence of the *Sozial Demokratische Partei* among workers in the new Germany. Meanwhile Rudolf Virchow had already published *Die Medizinische Reform* in 1848, following a request by the Prussian Ministry of Health, concluding that the most serious diseases were associated with social problems and therefore medical action had to be closely linked to political action. Similarly, Max von Pettenkofer's surveys on health economics in Bavaria, *Über die Wert der Gesundheit für eine Stadt* (1873), outlined the financial benefits of investing in health and sanitation. Thus health was very much part of the Body Politic.[18]

In the interwar period, international health organisations became increasingly important both in policy formation and knowledge circulation. There were, however, organised efforts to make knowledge and ideas circulate also in earlier periods, as demonstrated in Guillem's chapter on food security, and that French paediatrics and child health policies became an inspiration for many European countries is well known from previous research.[19]

A European perspective shows a close relationship between rural health programmes and the structure of the public health administration in each country: within different traditions, there was often a close relationship between local and state levels of action. In the case of rural health institutions, for example, Tore Grønlie shows that 'local ownership' was an important concept, in that health institutions contributed to and became part of local identity, with feelings of belonging to a community and of having certain rights there. This seems to be an essential factor to acknowledge in the making of local and/or national identities more generally during the historical period under review.

---

17 Sigerist, H.E. 'From Bismarck to Beveridge. Developments and Trends in Social Security Legislation', *Bulletin of the History of Medicine, 13*, (1943), 365-388. See Hamlin, C. *Public Health and Social Justice in the Age of Chadwick*, Cambridge, Cambridge University Press, 1998.

18 Rosen, G. 'Economic and Social Policy in the Development of Public Health. An Essay in Interpretation', *Journal of the History of Medicine and Allied Sciences, 8,* (1953), 406-430. See Berg, M. and Cocks, G. (eds.) *Medicine and Modernity. Public Health and Medical Care in 19th and 20th Century Germany*, Cambridge, Cambdrige University Press, 1997.

19 Perdiguero Gil, E. (comp.) *Salvad al niño. Estudios sobre la protección a la infancia en la Europa mediterránea a comienzos del siglo XX,* Valencia, PUV/SEC, 2004.

Sources and approaches

Approaching these issues at a European level implies that a plurality of sources have been used, including legal regulations, local and national records, local archives, administrative publications and technical reports, medical topographies, religious and military archives, according to proactive or reactive orientations. We hope that the volume can serve as an inspiration to further research and offer some guidelines as to relevant sources below and in the select bibliography.

In a recent issue of *Dynamis,* E. Rodríguez Ocaña anticipates the enhanced importance of rural health research in the history of medicine, suggesting that, in addition to the question of sources, a primary challenge will be to combine local and comparative, specific orientations with more integrative or systematic approaches. Meanwhile, in this introduction we have offered some perspectives of rural health that might serve to illuminate why rural health became an issue in Europe and, furthermore, illustrate the different research approaches adopted by the volume's contributors.[20]

Two overarching themes have emerged from our studies. The first concerns shifting images of 'The rural', from clean and healthy to a breeding ground for contagious and culture-bound diseases. This requires analysis of changing perceptions of rural health; the medical contributions to these shifts; the contexts in which they occurred and continuing ambiguity surrounding the rural where sickness and health were concerned. A second theme is the increasing political importance of public health everywhere – not just in urban areas – and the attempted provision of health care or specific services to all, rather than only to town dwellers or those able to afford doctoring and amenities. An understated element in this process is the extent to which European comparisons served as a political tool for states and medical authorities: health policies served to position each nation state among other states, indicating strengths or weaknesses, increasingly refining earlier mercantilist views focused upon population numbers rather than health.

The volume underscores the well-known point that poverty is an enemy of good health. However, it also reveals the extent to which poverty has been defined as a cultural question and it investigates different understandings about sickness among rural populations. It highlights the intricate association of cultural habits and living standards; the sometimes strained relationship between science and politics; and the deliberate measures taken by authorities of differing political complexion to 'civilise' and 'modernise' rural societies in the name of health, population quality and international competition. Notions of rights and citizenship were increasingly invoked over time, though more prominently

---

20 *Dynamis, 28*, (2008), 457-460

under democratic than authoritarian rule. While the importance of political systems – and political cultures – upon health services offered to populations is demonstrated, the influence of 'the rural' upon health policies and of rural epidemiological features upon medical science are key questions addressed here. Examples of failed or underdeveloped projects as well as successes are considered, taking specific measures or innovations within the overall contexts that made for improvements or otherwise in standards of rural health and hygiene.

TRACHOMA, HEALTH CONDITIONS AND SOCIAL CHANGE IN SARDINIA

Paola M. Melis and Lucia Pozzi

This chapter considers health conditions among the Sardinian rural population from the time of National Unification in 1861 through the first half of the twentieth century, focusing upon trachoma, a disease strongly conditioned by environmental, sanitary and socio-economic factors. It concentrates on two specific communities: Alghero, a small port located along the north western coast, and the villages of Talana and Urzulei, situated in the central-eastern region of the island called Ogliastra. Alghero was a semi-rural small town and Talana and Urzulei were remote, tiny rural villages. We examine the fight against trachoma in these different contexts, taking into account also related developments in the urban provincial capitals.[1] We outline the widespread trachoma prevalence in different areas of Sardinia noting urban and rural differentials in its eventual eradication. We address the interplay of legislation, its implementation moving from urban to rural areas, the role of education and of improving social conditions in overcoming this disease.

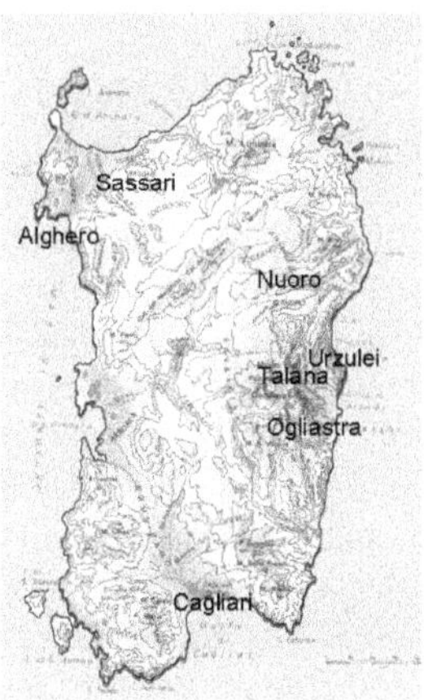

Trachoma is mentioned in ancient Egyptian papyrus texts and in early Chinese writings. It remains a worldwide problem: from seven to ten million people are blinded and up to 84 million are affected by it, according to the 2002 World Health Organisation estimates.[2] In developed countries it disappeared during the twentieth century. In 1907 *Chlamydia trachomatis*, the bacterium that causes trachoma, was first identified and in 1957 it was cultured *in vitro*. Serological diagnostic tests, developed in the 1930s, became more sophisticated and precise in the 1970s. Trachoma treatment evolved from ancient Egyptian usage of animal, vegetable and mineral products applied to the eyes using feathers, to the classical Greek physicians' methods of scarification of the granular

1 At the time of national unification, the island was divided in two provinces: Sassari in the North and Cagliari (the island's capital) in the South. Alghero was part of the northern province while Talana and Urzulei were part of Cagliari until 1927 when Nuoro province was created.

2 Taylor, H. *Trachoma: A Blinding Scourge from the Bronze Age to the Twenty-first century,* East Melbourne, Victoria, Centre for Eye Research, Australia, Haddington Press, 2008.

conjunctiva, followed by application of copper compounds and surgical excision of the fleshy granular tissue of the lids to correct entropion and trichiasis.[3] The latter methods spread from the Middle East to Western medicine in the Middle Ages, remaining the basis of treatments until the introduction of the first reasonably effective antimicrobials, the sulphonamides in 1937, but tetracycline and other antibiotics are now widely used.

The persistence of trachoma in the poor areas of the world, its epidemiology and the frequency of re-infection even in presence of free antibiotics distribution, leads us to conclude that the pharmacological treatment of the disease is insufficient for complete eradication. Environmental and social conditions linked to poor living standards, lack of hygiene and cleanliness are factors in its treatment to be considered just as important as the medical possibility of effective cure.

Legislative measures adopted in Italy to fight trachoma

Mandatory reporting of infectious diseases was introduced under Italian legislation in 1888. A ministerial directive for public schools on April 1st 1892 requested the 'isolation of trachoma affected children in benches kept in a separate area of the classroom and the periodical presentation of medical certification proving the continuous treatment'.[4] In 1903 the Ministry of the Interior published a directive re-establishing similar rules as earlier measures had not produced the desired effects. Trachoma was highlighted as one 'long term disease, requiring that affected children under treatment would be admitted to special trachoma schools or, in their absence, to public schools but kept in separated classes or in secluded areas of the classrooms'. In 1905, and again in 1912, the Public Health General Manager directed provincial Prefects in high incidence areas to implement therapeutic measures to fight trachoma. The first free trachoma clinics and surgeries were created in most cities and courses were established at University Ophthalmological Clinics on its diagnosis, prophylaxis and cure for medical officers, general practitioners and private doctors. These directives formed the basis for the first direct attempt on the part of the Italian State to combat trachoma.[5]

Later, especially during the Fascist era (1922-43), further refining directives and ministerial decrees were issued. From 1919 the mandatory reporting of trachoma cases was extended to communities such as boarding schools, hospitals,

---

3 Bietti, G.B. *Il Tracoma*, Rome, Alto Commissariato per l'Igiene e la Sanità Pubblica, 1947.

4 Comune di Sassari, *Le Scuole Elementari, anni 1905-06, 1906-07, 1907-08. Relazione Generale*, Sassari, Premiato Stabilimento Tipografico Ditta G. Dessì, 1909.

5 Pintus, L. and Latte, B. 'Considerazioni sulla Lotta Antitracomatosa nella Popolazione Scolastica: Risultati conseguiti nelle colonie estive istituite dall'E.P.A. di Nuoro dal 1954 al 1959. Nota II', *L'Igiene Moderna*, LIII, n. 11-12. 1960.

orphanages, nurseries and day-care centres, prisons and factories. In 1921 a royal decree established that affected children should be removed from school until fully healed but, since cure could take a very long time, they could be re-admitted if 'there was no discharge associated to the inflammation'. Trachoma-affected adults were prohibited from employment in the preparation and sale of food and drink, and in the manufacture of milk and meat products.[6] The consolidation of sanitary laws in 1934 involved 'special measures of prophylaxis and assistance for some diseases in man', specifically tuberculosis, trachoma, venereal diseases and leprosy. Doctors were obliged to report any case coming under their attention, on penalty of fines. Ministry of Health funded walk-in clinics and university courses to treat and combat trachoma diffusion were enhanced by special financial aid for those municipalities that established special schools for trachoma-affected children.[7] However, funds for the enactment of the measures were always insufficient, especially for the smallest provincial towns and villages.

In 1939, trachoma remained unabated in 24 southern provinces of Italy and a Governmental Inquiry was established to analyse the situation and to propose a full remedial solution. Prof. Ruata, an ophthalmologist from Rome University, and Dr Campanella, a Ministry of Health specialist in Hygiene and Sanitary Policy, published their results in 1940. [8] Tracing the development of trachoma from infancy through to adulthood, they described how it became steadily more resistant and severe, especially in subjects weakened by other diseases or chronic malnourishment. Thus nursery and elementary schools were the most appropriate places to begin anti-trachoma measures, with affected children to be identified and separated from healthy children, and school dispensaries established to sustain the curative effort. School meals were to be provided for indigent children with special summer camps in areas with good climates established to restore them into good health. The report prompted the creation of an *Ente Provinciale Antitracomatoso* (EPA) in each of the 24 provinces, financed by State and public contributions, though the proposed measures remained in the realm of good intentions. EPA policy regulations were published and administrative structures created, but in 1940 when Italy entered World War Two the fight against trachoma was put on hold.

However, in the city of Sassari the EPA had already been created in 1931 by the Prefect, at the suggestion of the provincial medical officer and supported by

---

6 Bietti, *Il tracoma*, 106.

7 Royal Decree 27/07/1934, Number 1265.

8 Ruata, V. and Campanella, F. *Lo Stato Attuale di Diffusione del Tracoma nell'Italia Meridionale ed Insulare*, Rome, Istituto Poligrafico dello Stato, 1940.

the 'Sassari Committee for the fight against trachoma' founded in the 1920s.[9] Between 1931 and 1933 the Sassari EPA created 84 new dispensaries in the provincial centres. In 1945 the Alto Commissariato per l'Igiene e la Sanità (ACIS) was created with financial support from the United Nations Relief and Rehabilitation Administration (UNRRA), promoting the establishment of numerous dispensaries, differential classes and summer camps for affected children.

Alghero, Talana and Urzulei

Sardinia after Unification had a very poor economy, typically based on agriculture, sheep-farming, fishery and mining. Around 1900 almost two thirds of the male population was occupied in these activities, and still 55 per cent in 1921. Cultivations were traditionally limited to olives, vines, fruits, cereals and legumes. Farming, including dairying, was small scale and non-technological with poor and unprofitable products.[10] Low population density was characteristic of Sardinia, with just 26 inhabitants per sq km – the lowest in Italy – compared to the national average of 91, and this situation remained unchanged.[11]

Alghero, a little coastal town of Catalan origin, was the third largest municipality of the province of Sassari, with 8,419 inhabitants in 1861, rising to 12,510 in 1921.[12] The municipal territory to the north included the Nurra plain, the only true 'scattered habitat area' of the region, according to the famous French geographer Maurice Le Lannou.[13] The presence of 100 hectares of stagnant brackish water favoured the spread of malaria, greatly affecting popular health. Marriage records confirm the predominance of agriculture in the male occupational structure, as in the rest of the island, but also maritime activities, with 15-20 per cent of grooms classified as 'sailors' or 'fishermen'.

Sardinia was characterised by a lack of roads and railways and communications across the island were always very poor. Because of the sea and the harbour, Alghero had more outside contacts, which helped to develop the local economy, favouring small industrial activities at the end of the nineteenth century. But isolation, poverty, and absence of interaction with the mainland had

9 Provincia di Sassari, Ente Provinciale per la lotta contro il tracoma, *Statuto e regolamento*, Sassari, Stamperia della Libreria Italiana e Straniera, 1932.

10 Coda L. *La Sardegna nella crisi di fine secolo. Aspetti dell'economia e della società sarda nell'ultimo ventennio dell'Ottocento*, Sassari, Editrice Libreria Dessì, 1977.

11 Satta Dessolis, A. *Dati e Considerazioni sul Problema Demografico in Sardegna*, Siena, Circolo Giuridico della R. Università, 1933.

12 The two major cities of the province were the capital, Sassari, and Tempio. Nowadays Alghero population is about 40,000.

13 Le Lannou, M. *Pastori e contadini di Sardegna*, 4th Italian Edition (M. Brigaglia transl. of *Pâtres et paysans de la Sardaigne*, Tours, Arrault, 1941), Cagliari, Edizioni Della Torre, 2006.

dire consequences on the general level of education of the Sardinian population. In the 1881 census over 75 per cent of the island population aged above six years was still illiterate and Alghero had 73 per cent illiterate inhabitants. Before 1900 most people lived in the historic centre, enclosed by the Catalan walls, where sanitary and hygienic conditions featured 'alarming' levels of water contamination and open air sewers, according to a national sanitary inspection.[14] Another national survey of Italian municipalities in 1885, following a destructive cholera outbreak, confirmed the dismal conditions in Alghero, noting deficient hygienic infrastructures and undrinkable water. However, there were six doctors, three pharmacists and three registered midwives active in town and the municipal administration had a contract with the local hospital, administered by the *Congregazione della Carità,* for the cure of indigent citizens.[15] In 1910, 956 families were classified as 'indigent', constituting roughly one-third of the total population according to the municipal government, which estimated an average family size of four.

The Ogliastra region in east-central Sardinia represented 'an island in the island' because of its isolation and geographical seclusion, bounded by mountains and a very rocky coastline except for the Tortolì harbour. [16] As the plains around Tortolì were marshy and affected by malaria until the late 1950s, most Ogliastra villages were built on mountainsides between 400 and 800 metres above sea level. Ogliastra had, in 2001, almost 58,400 inhabitants and comprises 23 villages varying in size today from 500 to 10,000 inhabitants, with the lowest population density of the entire country: 31.7 inhabitants per square kilometre, below the regional average of 67.7 and far below the national average of 194.

The Government Inquiry into the Italian agrarian population in the late 1870s described Ogliastra as one of the poorest and most under-developed areas, even by Sardinian standards. It underlined the backwardness of the entire agrarian productive system and the almost complete lack of commercialisation of local products.[17] Only cheese production was particularly abundant in the area but this

---

14 Casu, P. M. *Relazione della Visita Sanitaria eseguita nel 1860 nel circondario di Alghero dal chimico farmacista Pietro Maria Casu*, Turin, 1860.

15 Ministero di Agricoltura, Industria e Commercio (MAIC), Direzione generale della Statistica (Dirstat), *Risultati dell'inchiesta sulle condizioni igienico sanitarie dei comuni del Regno. Relazione Generale*, Rome, Tipografia nell'Ospizio di San Michele, 1886.

16 La Marmora, A. *Itinerario dell'Isola di Sardegna.* Italian Edition (Longhi, M. G. transl. of *Itinéraire de l'Ile de Sardaigne, pour faire suite au Voyage en cette contrée*, tome I-II, Turin, Fréres Bocca, 1860) 3 volumes, Nuoro, Ilisso Edizioni, 1997.

17 Rivera-Ricci, A. 'Sull'Organismo Agrario del Circondario di Lanusei. Monografia Agraria', part of 'Relazione del Commissario Francesco Salaris sulla XII circoscrizione (Sardegna)', in *Atti della Giunta per l'Inchiesta Agraria e sulle Condizioni della Classe Agricola.* Vol. XIV, Rome, Forzani e C. Tipografi del Senato, 1882.

was still done in artisanal fashion and for local consumption.[18] The great extension of communal territories maintained two traditional and ancient systems of common land use which had already disappeared in other Sardinian areas. First, the vidazzone system regimented rules and turns in the use of certain parcels of land to resolve the diverging interests of farmers and shepherds and, second, common land was attributed to resident families according to the ancient Roman law of emphyteusis, which involved the obligation to make improvements to increase the value of the land. [19] These systems restricted nineteenth century enclosure laws and prevented the formation of large estates, thus maintaining local populations.

This was a world where five-year old children were tending animals, carrying firewood and fetching water. National laws for mandatory public primary education dating from 1859 were not enforceable because of lack of schools and teachers and the general poverty of municipalities responsible for education, health care and other tasks associated with state rules and public administration. The 1890 Government Health Inquiry lamented that 'both pregnant women and small children worked like animals in the fields' and, as a consequence, children showed pathological signs of deficient organic development, including bone deformations and deviation of the vertebral column.[20] Many of these aspects of mountain life extended beyond World War Two as improvements were very slow in reaching this extreme periphery of Sardinia.[21]

In the 1861 census Talana had 448 inhabitants and Urzulei 579, increasing respectively to 763 and 1,026 in 1921.[22] The general level of poverty was attested by the 'list of indigent people' having the right to free medical assistance prepared yearly by the municipal administration. The number fluctuated considerably, reflecting the application of different directives from above or the contingency of municipal budgets, rather than changes in status. Moreover, the villages lacked decent roads and necessary infrastructures (cemetery, sewage system, aqueduct, elementary and nursery school buildings) until the 1950s.

---

18 As a consequence, there was almost no circulation of money. Almost all transactions were based on barter and even rural labourers received payment in kind as late as the 1940s. One of the first significant inputs of money came from the war pensions received by the heirs of fallen soldiers in World War One.

19 The vidazzone system was abandoned when emigration started in the 1960s while the system of emphyteusis is still in place since the leased land can be inherited if conditions are respected.

20 Panizza, M. *Risultati dell'inchiesta istituita da Agostino Bertani sulle condizioni sanitarie dei lavoratori della terra in Italia: riassunto e considerazioni*, Rome, Stabilimento Tipografico Italiano, 1890.

21 Since 1995 the inhabitants of Talana ans Urzulei have participated in a multidisciplinary research project on the identification of genes predisposing to common complex diseases.

22 In the last census (2001) Talana had a population of 1,129 inhabitants and Urzulei 1,443.

All this undermined the possibility of effective medical care, whether for the indigent or the 'better off' citizens. The archives of both villages reflect continual efforts to secure the services of general practitioners by forming joint consortiums in order to save money. These regularly failed and each village then tried to hire its own doctor but was unable to attract or retain one. The contracted doctors came from Dorgali or Baunei, about 25 km away from Urzulei (one north and the other south of this village), with Talana 15 km further to the west. Spending one day a week in each village, doctors could not attend to local needs.[23] Around 1900 the only hospital in the province was in Nuoro. Founded in 1883 as *Pia Opera dello Spedale San Francesco*, it was actually constructed some 20 years later on municipal land with philanthropic support from local rich families. In 1933 it had only a surgical service, and offered 30 beds for a provincial population of 220,000. Plans to enlarge it revealed that, in 1933, ophthalmic patients were refused hospitalisation if contagious (as in the case of seriously ill trachoma patients) because there was no 'isolation ward'.[24] The frequent lack of doctors and the distances involved in seeking medical care was reflected in the many permanent injuries incurred by children and young adults, as revealed by physical examinations during conscription: limb fractures and dislocations improperly treated or not treated at all left many young men maimed and unfit for military service.[25]

Poverty and diseases in the populations under study

Poor health and dismal hygienic conditions in Italy were described in numerous late nineteenth-century Governmental inquiries.[26] At the same time, military data confirmed high levels of temporary or permanent rejections of young men at call-up visits, but this problem was at its most dramatic for the Sardinian youths. Giuseppe Sormani (1881), in research based on cohorts born 1843-56 for all the Italian military districts, documented the dire health situation and prevalence of diseases of different origins.[27] He was particularly caustic about

23 Often months passed before a new doctor would be found after the resignation of one. The signatures on death certificates and the deliberations for a new doctor nomination, attest the extremely frequent turnover of medical doctors in these villages. Between 1907 and 1962 Urzulei had 43 different doctors. Talana had about the same turnover. Things changed for Talana in the late 1950s and in 1962 for Urzulei, when each obtained its own general practitioner. Furthermore, in 1956 a registered midwife was contracted by both villages and she remained in service until the 1980s.

24 Nuoro State Archive (ASNU), Fondo Prefettura, cat XIX, busta n. 132

25 ASNU, Draft Registers Circondario Lanusei

26 MAIC, Dirstat, *Risultati dell'inchiesta sulle condizioni igienico sanitarie dei comuni del Regno*; Panizza, *Risultati dell'inchiesta istituita da Agostino Bertani*.

27 The highest percentages were reached in Lombardy and in Sardinia, but while in the first one the main reasons of permanent discharge were specific diseases as well as insufficient

Sardinia, commenting that, of 1,000 conscripts there, it was impossible to 'dig out' more than 400 soldiers. A particular characteristic was insufficient height: whereas the Italian average for individuals so rejected was 13.1 per cent, in Sardinia it was 27.4 per cent and in some *trachoma Circondari* was much higher, notably in Alghero with 30 per cent and Lanusei, highest of all, with 43.8 per cent.

We have examined the military draft lists, collecting all recorded data for the community of Alghero for the cohorts born between 1866 and 1900, and similarly for the Ogliastra region for the same cohorts at a five years cadence, with additional focus on two districts (Lanusei and Tortolì) which include the municipalities of Talana and Urzulei. Each commune provided an annual list of males aged 20 years and those identified for call-up had to undergo anthropometric measurements in which height and thoracic circumference determined a preliminary elimination of below-standards youths. The others underwent medical examinations by military doctors or clinical specialists and were assessed as 'fit', 'unfit' or 'temporarily unfit' for military service. These sources refer only to the male population but this serial documentation provides us with sanitary and anthropometric indicators, elaborated by qualified personnel, and can be considered representative of the health situation of each Italian municipality.

The main results from our analysis can be summarised as follows:

a. Very high percentages of individuals were permanently or temporarily discharged, beyond most other Italian regions. In Alghero, 31 per cent of the male youths were classified as unfit for military service and another 31 per cent were temporarily unfit.[28] In the Ogliastra region they fared even worse, with 37.2 per cent unfit and 26.7 per cent temporarily unfit in Lanusei and in Tortolì district 35.1 per cent and 29.6 per cent respectively.
b. Insufficient height or thoracic circumference were the most prevalent reasons for permanent discharge. In Alghero and Tortolì districts about 70

height or insufficient thoracic circumference, in the island the most relevant reason for permanent discharge was insufficient height. See Sormani, G., 'Geografia nosologica d'Italia', Ministero Agricoltura, Industria e Commercio (MAIC), Direzione Generale di Statistica (Dirstat), *Annali di Statistica*, serie II, vol. VI. 1881.

28 These are the average percentages recorded for the male cohorts born between 1866-1900, for more detailed information see Cau, P.; Merella, C.; Pozzi, L. 'Lo stato di salute della popolazione di Alghero fra '800 e '900. Uno studio condotto attraverso i registri militari', in Breschi, M. and Pozzi, L. (eds.) *Salute, malattia e sopravvivenza in Italia fra '800 e '900*, Udine, Forum, 135-56, 2007.

per cent of military rejections were due to insufficient height, while in Lanusei district the percentage was 78 per cent.

c. Very low mean heights and thoracic circumferences before 1916 with no significant modifications over time. The mean height for Alghero was about 159 cm. while in Tortoli and Lanusei it was respectively 157 and 156 cm. The mean thoracic circumferences were 82 cm. for Alghero, 81 and 80 for Tortolì and Lanusei.
d. Strong socio-economic differentials in the parametric indicators, with a difference of more than 7 cm. between the mean height of the poorest social category and the highest in the Alghero data.
e. Very high diffusion of malaria and ophthalmic diseases, in particular conjunctivitis and trachoma. In Lanusei district malaria caused 13 per cent of temporary discharges, with 30 per cent in Tortolì district, and about 11 per cent in Alghero. The relevance of ophthalmic diseases was particularly striking in Alghero, accounting for 34 per cent of temporary discharges, while in the districts of Lanusei and Tortolì the corresponding figures were five per cent and eight per cent.[29]

Various studies have presented height evolution as a valid proxy of population health or, more generally, an indicator of well-being.[30] The relationship of health and height involves a complex interplay of factors but, in these populations, short heights, even if influenced by genetic causes, reflected a high deprivation status.[31] Numerous early twentieth-century medical surveys also reported on the predominance of malaria, tuberculosis and trachoma in particular, throughout Sardinia, with high levels of deprivation and poor hygienic standards as the

29 A recent study has confirmed a higher frequency of ophthalmic diseases in Sardinia, causing permanent or temporary discharge, in comparison with other Italian regions. See Bussini, O. and Lanari, D. 'Statura e condizioni di salute della popolazione maschile a fine Ottocento: uno studio basato sui registri di leva', in Breschi and Pozzi (eds.) *Salute, malattia e sopravvivenza*, 105-33.

30 See Tanner, J.M. 'Growth as a measure of the nutritional and hygienic status of a population', *Hormone Research*, 38 (Suppl.1), 1992, 106-115; Komlos, J. 'The secular trend in biological standard of living in the United Kingdom, 1730-1866', *Economic History Review*, XLVI, 1993, 115-144; Federico, G. 'Heights, calories and welfare: a new perspective on Italian industrialization, 1854-1913', *Economics and Human Biology*, 1, 2003, 289-308; Gatti A. M.; Calò C.M.; Piras I. S. 'Lo stato di salute delle leve militari in Sardegna tra Ottocento e Novecento'. In Corsini C.A. (ed.) *Statura, salute e migrazioni: le leve militari italiane*. Udine, Forum, 2008, 169-191.

31 Coletti emphasised that Sardinian conscripts grew more during military service than the rest of Italian soldiers. He wrote: 'Sardinian soldiers grow more than the others because they find in military life much better food, housing, hygiene and cures than they had in their villages'. See Coletti, F. *La mortalità nei primi anni di vita e la vita sociale della Sardegna*, Torino, Fratelli Bocca, 1908, 188.

main underlying features.[32] The 1885 National Survey had found that 'Blindness in Sardinia is so widespread compared to other regions that we have to postulate stronger causes that go beyond the geographical factors, like social conditions (i.e. poor hygiene, eye diseases frequency, myopia, smallpox etc.)'.[33] Twenty years later, Coletti identified trachoma as the main reason for blindness in the island, the 'region with the highest number of blind people in the Kingdom of Italy'. Whereas in 1872 there were 193 blind people per 100,000 inhabitants in Sardinia compared to 105 in Italy; in 1905 there were respectively 325 and 118.[34]

As we emphasise below, trachoma was directly linked by contemporary physicians with poverty and deprivation. For example, in 1923 Debenedetti wrote: 'This is why the fight against trachoma is also a social problem, the problem of indigence: the higher the standard of living, the lower the risk of contagion'.[35] Earlier, Coletti reported: 'Dr. E.A. from Sassari sends me the following information: the majority of blindness cases in Sardinia happen as a consequence of trachoma complications. Trachoma is very frequent in Sassari province, especially in Alghero and in other filthy villages, less so in hillside villages, where there are also fewer infectious diseases'.[36] As we shall see, the hill villages in Ogliastra contradict this statement: moreover, the shortness of young men implied that they were rejected at draft time without ever undergoing a medical examination, which suggests under-reporting of trachoma and other diseases here.[37]

---

32 Debenedetti, S. 'Diffusione del Tracoma nella città di Sassari', *Studi Sassaresi*, serie II vol. II (1925), 1-19; Maggiore, L. *Per combattere il tracoma nella città e nella provincia di Sassari. Problemi da risolvere e provvedimenti urgenti da attuare*, Sassari, Tip. Libreria Italiana e Straniera, 1926; Maggiore, L. 'Il Tracoma nella città e provincia di Sassari. Diffusione della malattia ed organizzazione delle opere di assistenza e profilassi sociale', *Studi Sassaresi*, Vol. IV, fasc. I, (1928), 527-576; Corbia, A. 'La mortalità per tubercolosi nella provincia di Sassari. Resoconto critico statistico per gli anni 1926-30', *Studi Sassaresi*, serie II vol. XII, Fasc. II. 1934; Collari S. *Il problema tubercolare sardo*, Rome, Federazione nazionale fascista per la lotta contro la tubercolosi, Stabilimento tipografico Europa, 1935; Pergola, A. *Le condizioni igieniche delle scuole elementari della provincia di Sassari in rapporto alle diffusione delle malattie oculari*, Sassari, Tipografia Gallizzi, 1935.

33 MAIC, Dirstat, *Risultati dell'inchiesta sulle condizioni igienico sanitarie dei comuni del Regno* 1886, XCX.

34 Coletti, *La mortalità nei primi anni di vita*, 87.

35 Debenedetti, 'Diffusione del Tracoma nella città di Sassari', 16.

36 Coletti, *La mortalità nei primi anni di vita*, 87.

37 During the last years of World War One, in the drive to increase the number of fighting soldiers, the height limits were decreased and all the previously 'rejected' youths were re-examined. In special military registers called *Riformati rivisitati* we find numerous previously rejected men being drafted even if 'affected by trachoma' and assigned to the 'trachoma battalion' of the 'Sassari Brigade' (ASNU, Draft Registers, 1915-1918).

We now focus upon the diffusion of trachoma and the sanitary campaign against it in the two areas analysed, beginning with Alghero.

The Alghero experience: the diffusion of trachoma and the fight against the disease

In official reports or medical publications on trachoma, Sassari province had the highest incidence in Italy and special attention was paid to Alghero:

> 'Trachoma, called also 'phylloxera of the eyes' because of its destructive action, is a serious social scourge as malaria and tuberculosis for the greatest part of the population of this province, which has the sad primacy among the other Italian provinces. It is extremely common in populous centres: Sassari had in the past 20% of its population affected, while in Alghero a fourth of the entire population was found affected.'[38]

However, it is far more difficult to review accurately the situation and counter-measures in Alghero than in the provincial capital, Sassari, where there was a University Ophthalmology Clinic. For example, in 1901 the Sassari municipal administration expelled from its elementary schools about 200 children affected by the disease in order to protect its healthy students and the elementary school director noted in 1900 that, out of 2,280 enrolled students, 107 boys and 121 girls were affected by trachoma. In response the municipal administration created the first 'trachoma school' with 405 students admitted. Of these, 289 were children of farmers, day labourers or porters, with 272 also admitted to the school lunch programme.[39] Sassari school registers confirmed that, in the period 1908-1913, the percentage of children affected fluctuated between 11.3 per cent and 14.8 per cent, far above levels in other Italian cities.[40] The situation actually worsened in the 1920s before it improved during the 1930s.

Maggiore, a Professor of Ophthalmology at the University of Sassari, observed the geography of the disease: it was worst among the poorest people living in the crowded part of the old town centre, whereas the newer middle-class

38 Sassari Provincial Archive (APSS), 1928, Sanità n. 11731.

39 The director of Sassari Elementary school, in a report to the Mayor, with dismay, annotated that in the school year 1907-08, the city of Sassari had not spent for each enrolled student, as much as the city of Milan had invested fifty years earlier, in the school year 1859-60. See Comune di Sassari, *Le Scuole Elementari*, 27

40 This was the situation in other Italian cities: Milan (5.0%), Padua (0.07%), Genoa (1.0%) and Bologna (1.5%) See Sotgia, G. M. *Il tracoma nelle scuole elementari di Sassari: relazione all'on amministrazione comunale nel 1913*, Sassari, Tipografia Operaia, 1921; Delogu, S. *Storia di una Malattia Sociale: il Tracoma in Sardegna dal 1900 al 1950*, Tesi di Laurea. Facoltà di Giurisprudenza, Corso di Laurea in Scienze Politiche. (Relatore Prof. Manconi F.), Università degli Studi di Sassari, 1990-91.

districts beyond were practically immune from the disease. However, he summarised the living conditions facing 90 per cent of the provincial population: 'Narrow hovels, with low roofs, often windowless, below ground level, with uneven or untiled floors, decaying walls, often with a sort of latrine in a corner of the single room'.[41] He also denounced the frequent use of one bed for the entire family; insufficient blankets replaced by old clothes; overcrowding and the lack of air, light and water: 'all of these are missing: 50 to 80 per cent of what is needed in the case of air and light, often 100 per cent in the case of water'.[42] Similar observations were still being recorded thirty years later in Nuoro province. Elsewhere, Maggiore found that:

> 'It is almost impossible to obtain complete and accurate data in order to identify all individuals affected by trachoma, because part of the population lives in the countryside and therefore out of reach of medical supervision, another part, even if affected, renounces or even voluntarily gives up the search for sanitary assistance.'[43]

That the 'rurals' were 'out of reach of medical supervision' suggests a situation of actual neglect of these populations (as attested below by the experience of Talana and Urzulei) due to various contingent reasons such as difficult access, lack of financial means and poor organisation. In fact dispensaries were mostly organised in larger population centres and Maggiore reported on their findings. In Alghero, of 694 people visiting the ophthalmological dispensary between 1925-27, 596 were affected by trachoma, or 85.8 per cent. However, the very lack of regular and continuous data referring to Alghero can be read as a sign of inadequate concern on the part of the authorities or, at least, of the insufficient resources available to prevent trachoma's spread in the absence of curative measures. As in the Ogliastra case, this documentary 'silence' speaks volumes about the neglect of the disease until the post-1945 era for Talana and Urzulei.

The Alghero school registers examined from 1901 suggest that attention was first paid to the problem of trachoma in public schools in 1905. From then on two ledgers were kept for each class: one containing information about students and teachers and the other with records of attendance, votes, examinations and final reports. The first ledger included teachers' comments on children, including those affected by trachoma that were removed from school by 'health official's order' and did not return that year. For 1908-09 and 1909-10 some registers were marked 'first grade - trachoma affected' or contain teachers' comments to that effect. There are no further notes until 1915 when a sheet containing a detailed medical diagnosis next to each name indicated an accurate medi-

---

41 Maggiore, *Per combattere il tracoma nella città e nella provincia di Sassari*, 4.
42 Maggiore, *Per combattere il tracoma*, 5
43 Maggiore, 'Il Tracoma nella città e provincia di Sassari', 526.

cal inspection.[44] Evidently there were no clear directives in Alghero schools for the identification of special classes until 1928, the beginning of the fascist strongest 'propaganda' phase.[45] A new format of 'Class Journals' required detailed information on planned academic programmes, month by month chronicles and observations on school life, and a report that each teacher should send to the school director at the end of the academic year. Trachoma classes are clearly marked, with teachers' chronicles offering glimpses into school life, the social conditions of the children attending the different classes, and painful details concerning trachoma-affected children and their backgrounds.[46]

Gaps in this data, the loss of registers or missing trachoma class labels affect the series we have reconstructed, but Table 1 illustrates how from one-quarter to one-third of first and second grade enrolled children were affected by the disease until the 1930s. Subsequently disease prevalence fluctuated, falling below ten per cent in the 1940s. First grade classes had the highest number of attending children and therefore also of those in the special trachoma classes. Comparing the Alghero school data with the series reconstructed for the city of Sassari, the results are very similar or somewhat higher in Alghero.[47]

---

44 The 1901 Sanitary Regulation Law n. 45 prescribed that the municipal health officer should visit the schools at least once a month, and the 1904 new regulation increased the visits to twice a month. See Comune di Sassari, *Le scuole elementari*, 57.

45 School registers is a rich information source on teachers and children attitudes. Schools became the main avenue of 'fascistizzazione' of the new generations. All the teachers were required to become members of the party and in the registers we find references to their efforts to collect party's dues from all the children and criticism towards the parents who do not have money to pay for them. School programmes reflect the party's myths creation and the religious imprinting pushed on the children. Sassari State Archive (ASSS), Alghero school registers, 1921-1943.

46 In 1928 the first grade trachoma-class teacher Caterina De Giorgio, in her final report used almost poetic terms to describe her class: 'my students were very poor, sick, unhappy children. They were the street child, the nobody's child, the panhandler's child, the wretch that fights with hunger, the beggar that picks up the rich kid's left-over.' Some teachers were dismayed by the assignment, as Assunta Mela who, in October 1934, writes 'the director could not play a worse trick on me by moving me from a regular first grade to a 'trachoma third grade'. But later on she feels pity for her students 'After the cure the children suffer a lot' and she allowed them to put the head down on the table (ASSS, Alghero school registers).

47 For the data about the city of Sassari see Sotgia, 'Il tracoma nelle scuole elementari'; De Benedetti, 'Diffusione del tracoma nella città di Sassari'; Pergola, A. *Rilievi sociali e clinici sulla lotta antitracomatosa in provincia di Sassari e risultati ottenuti nel quinquennio 1932-37*, Turin, Tipografia e Litografia Carlo Accame, 1937.

Table 1 Alghero: enrolled and trachoma-affected children in elementary first and second grades (1908-1937)

School year	Enrolled	Trachoma	%	School year	Enrolled	Trachoma	%
1908-09	416	139	33.4	1926-27			
1909-10	464	95	20.5	1927-28			
1910-11	342			1928-29			
1911-12	407			1929-30	472	99	21.0
1912-13	514			1930-31	339	93	27.4
1913-14	435			1931-32	543	165	30.4
1914-15	513			1932-33	434	110	25.3
1915-16	477	98	20.5	1933-34	554	140	25.3
1915-17				1934-35	490	53	10.8
1917-18				1935-36	558	93	16.7
1918-19				1936-37	539	64	11.9
1919-20	558			1937-38	607	126	20.8
1920-21	496			1938-39		95	
1921-22	511			1939-40	463		
1922-23	563	98	17.4	1940-41	619	47	7.6
1923-24				1941-42	541	45	8.3
1924-25				1942-43	542	29	5.4

Sources: ASSS, Alghero School Registers

Documents classified as the 'Fight against trachoma' in the Alghero Municipal archive attest long and difficult procedures in organising the municipal anti-trachoma dispensaries and other initiatives. Although the city and provincial administration of Sassari had been prominent in anti-trachoma efforts, progress elsewhere was limited and slow.[48] The Fascist regime in the 1920s and 1930s ran a major propaganda campaign in the city, involving leaflets, university courses for health professionals and teachers, public notices and the clergy. Yet the rest of the province was hindered by inadequate funds and insufficient coordination among state, provincial and municipal authorities. For example, the 1901 Sanitary Regulations Newsletter requiring notification of trachoma cases, which led to the creation of a trachoma school in Sassari, was evidently transmitted to the Alghero municipal administration only on March 23rd 1915.[49] The impression gained from these records is that peripheral municipalities were

48 At the beginning of the twentieth century two anti trachoma surgeries were already functioning in the city of Sassari. In 1914 three school dispensaries were instituted in the elementary schools of the most affected areas. In 1925 a third surgery for the treatment of the general population was opened on the basis of the presence of 6,000 affected people out of a population of 44,000 inhabitants. Then, in 1932, three more clinics were opened, bringing the total number of trachoma clinics in the city to 6, plus the school dispensaries. See Delogu, *Storia di una Malattia Sociale*.

49 Such communications could have been sent before or were not saved but, in cases of repeated appeals, provincial authorities conventionally cited all previous correspondence.

aware of the environmental and health problems afflicting the populations but lacked the financial means to address them or sufficient support from overseeing bureaucratic structures: state officials were in distant cities and had little respect for rural representatives. Each had different realities: limited financial means and the need to 'make do' on one side, compared with strict 'by the book' rules and regulations, lacking flexibility or understanding, on the other.

For example, in May 1914 Alghero's Mayor, encouraged by Antonio Luigi Sotgiu, a Sardinian ophthalmologist living and practicing in Rome, informed the Sassari Prefect that the municipal administration intended to create a trachoma clinic during the summer months. It would provide rooms, equipment, furniture and medications, but he requested a 2,000 lira operating contribution.[50] Though pleased by this, the Prefect nevertheless refused since 'State subsidies are planned only for clinics to be established in provincial capitals'. Meanwhile the sub-Prefect advised the Mayor to proceed, since the Prefect might in future be able to request a State subsidy, so the clinic was organised, thanks to the free cooperation of Dr. Antonio Pisanu and a modest stipend for a male nurse paid by the township. Over time the clinic became part of the Hospital administered by the *Congregazione della Carità* but was always short of money and late in answering to the provincial authorities.[51] The Municipality also organised a dispensary in the elementary school and a special 22-bed trachoma isolation ward in the local hospital. Yet the State was hardly encouraging in its financial contributions: the first recorded payment of 1,500 liras being dated August 16th, 1923.[52]

No effective cures for trachoma were provided until 1939, when sulphonamide drugs were introduced throughout the Sassari province and provided free to patients and school children in dispensaries. Sulpha drugs actually limited the trachoma complications but did not eradicate the disease: after a decade tra-

---

50 In the voluminous correspondence relating to the establishment of this anti-trachoma clinic the 'necessity to find support in Rome through political contacts and personal recommendations' reflected a deplorable and widespread mentality still existing in Italy (ACA, 'Fight against trachoma').

51 The municipality decided on an annual contribution of 300 liras to the *Congregazione della carità*, starting in 1915, but in 1921 correspondence from the hospital was still soliciting these contributions. Alghero Municipal Archive (ACA), 'Fight against trachoma'.

52 Sassari provincial archive has documents relating to one year of anti-trachoma fight, signed by Professor Castello and dated September 27th, 1929, tracing also the new activities in Alghero where, from June 1929, an anti-trachoma 'house calls service' was instituted, with 272 families or 611 people inspected. Of these 437 were trachoma-affected but only 130 had received any previous treatment, 'incomplete and long ago interrupted'. The visiting doctor was accompanied by two specialised nurses, one of whom coming from Turin especially for this purpose. Meanwhile a new evening clinic and school dispensaries offered daily medications (APSS Sanità n. 11731).

choma still affected some 11 per cent of the population, though the incidence of complications had decreased from 65-70 per cent to 26 per cent during that time.[53] A study of draftees in Sassari 1900-1950 also concluded that trachoma morbidity had not decreased: 'After a decade of intense anti-trachoma struggle carried out in the entire province with sulpha drugs and antibiotics, trachoma frequency, after a false downturn during the war years (1940-45), had again reached the level it had in the years preceding the introduction of chemical therapeutics'.[54] Its higher prevalence in certain centres remained and among these was Alghero, 'where the greatest part of the population lives in overcrowded neighbourhoods with dismal hygienic conditions'.[55]

The fight against trachoma in Nuoro province

The Nuoro province was created in 1927 by subtracting areas from Cagliari and Sassari provinces and was the poorest province in Sardinia. In 1957 it ranked 88 out of the 92 Italian provinces in annual per capita income and it had the lowest level of literacy - 44.7 per cent of people with an elementary school education - throughout the 1950s. Its male and female working population aged ten years or over at the 1951 census was 43.3 per cent and, of these, 67.5 per cent were employed in agriculture, 14.7 per cent in industry and 8.2 per cent in commerce and services. Local industries included cheese making, wood cutting and mining with artisanal production of rugs, textiles, ceramics and baskets reaching a very restricted market.[56]

Around 1900 the percentage of trachoma cases in Nuoro province was not very high but the situation was deteriorating and a 1910 study of Nuoro district conscripts born between 1878 and 1887 showed increasing levels of trachoma.[57] This probably reflected the worsening economic, social and hygienic conditions in the district, as reflected in greater emigration from the area and, indeed, from all of Sardinia. In 1927, in Nuoro and six other towns with trachoma clinics, 988 of the 1,953 people visited were identified as trachoma affected. Some 344 required hospitalisation for complications but this was not possible since the San

---

53 Pasca C. 'Considerazioni statistiche sugli effetti della sulfamidoterapia del tracoma', *Bollettino di oculistica 1948*, cited by Delogu, *Storia di una Malattia Sociale*, 88.

54 Arghittu, C. 'Rilievi statistici su 168.000 iscritti di leva della provincia di Sassari appartenenti a 50 classi e visitati negli anni dal 1900 al 1950', *L'Igiene moderna*, Sassari, 1954, 679-680.

55 Arghittu, 'Rilievi statistici su 168.000 iscritti', 680.

56 Pintus, L. and Latte, B. 'Stato Attuale di Diffusione del Tracoma nella Provincia di Nuoro con Particolare Riguardo alla Popolazione Scolastica', *L'Igiene Moderna*, 53, n. 9-10. 1960, 527-551.

57 Marchi, F. A. *Il Tracoma nel Circondario di Nuoro*, Cagliari, Stabilimento Tipografico G. Montorsi, 1910.

Francesco Hospital in the provincial capital could not accept ophthalmic patients.[58] The same year inspections of 5,750 of the school population of 7,759 in Nuoro province found 7.8 per cent affected by trachoma.[59] After the 1940 Government Report on trachoma diffusion in southern Italy and the islands, the provincial authorities in Nuoro created an anti-trachoma board (EPA). Each municipality was required to contribute to this on the basis of its 1936 census population and, with key personnel appointed, the EPA prepared annual reports. However the war prevented deliveries of drugs or equipment; dispensaries failed to open and school inspections and summer camps did not take place.[60]

The Public Health General Manager was very critical of the Nuoro dispensaries' inaction and threatened disciplinary sanctions against the inspectors,

> 'whose duty it is to visit the most remote and smallest villages in the area in order to give advice to the non-specialist doctor, invested with the duty to fight trachoma and to report the efficiency of each dispensary. The inspector, moreover, should pay particular attention to the census of trachoma affected children in elementary schools. In the mean time he should, in agreement with the school superintendent, organise that special classes would be set up whenever there are more than 30 students affected by trachoma and insure that they would receive a convenient therapy with sulpha drugs in school dispensaries.'[61]

The EPA Rules and Regulations booklet established the duties of trachoma inspectors, clinic directors and visiting health assistants. Particular attention was given to completing forms for the municipal health officer containing the names of affected children identified in schools. Their family members were then identified and summoned for an ocular examination and the visiting health assistant would seek to convince non-compliants of the necessity to be examined by the specialist. No individual forms were found in the Nuoro State archive and very few monthly statistical summaries have survived but Table 2 below contains data for the whole province.[62]

---

58 ASNU, Fondo Prefettura, Gabinetto, Cat. XIX, busta n. 132.

59 Mura, F. 'Problemi Sociali Isolani: il Tracoma', *Mediterranea: Rivista mensile di cultura e problemi isolani*, 11-12, (1929), 7-13.

60 ASNU, Fondo Prefettura, EPA-Bilancio, years 1942; 1943; 1944.

61 ASNU, Fondo Prefettura, Atti amministrativi, busta n. 63, Cat. XV Sanità, 11/11/1942.

62 An Annex gave instruction on a modified MacCallan trachoma classification to be used in the compilation of individual and general forms: T1: seen typically soon after infection has occurred; T2: in which follicles predominate but can coexist with papillary hypertrophy and chronic conjunctivitis; T3: in which cicatrisation is forming; T4: in which cicatrisation is complete. ASNU, EPA, varie, 1.15.10 Nuoro folder, EPA regolamento-tipo per i servizi e per il personale degli Enti provinciali antitracomatosi, Roma, Istituto Poligrafico dello Stato, 1941.

The Nuoro State Archive conserves separate information on the antitrachoma campaign for 34 of the 99 municipalities in the province, mostly dating from the 1930s, when municipal health officers reported on the need for trachoma clinics in their respective centres. The prevalence of the disease among school children was extremely high, varying from 30 to 60 per cent, but no further information is given. Only in the 1950s were the EPA inspections actually started and more data collected. Inactivity and the 'do nothing policy' were exemplified by the tentative creation of a trachoma hospital in the town of Macomer, in Nuoro Province in 1945. It was to be built by the *Presidenza del Consiglio dei Ministri*, the *Istituto Superiore della Sanità* and the *Alto Commissariato per l'Igiene e la Sanità* (ACIS) with the international contribution of UNRRA using a former army barracks. In 1955, when the premises were finally ready and the budgeted expenses had practically tripled, the barracks were requisitioned again by the army and the entire enterprise was aborted.[63] Meanwhile, the EPAs examination of school children in the three Sardinian provinces for 1957-58 showed that the percentage affected had actually increased in Nuoro province in comparison with 1927.

Table 2 Elementary schools enrolled and trachoma affected children in Sardinian provinces (school year 1957-58)

Province	Primary school children	Trachoma affected children	Trachoma affected children %
Cagliari	94,036	3,291	3.5
Sassari	37,557	1,342	3.6
Nuoro	32,153	2,731	8.5
Total	163,746	7,364	4.5

Source: Pintus, L.; Latte, B., 'Stato Attuale di Diffusione del tracoma…', 531

A further inspection of all the elementary school children in 102 provincial towns, villages and sections in 1959-60 provided the following results, summarised in Table 3 according to the MacCallan classification, described in note 62.

Table 3 Trachoma examinations in Nuoro province elementary schools (1959-60)

Total children visited	Total cases	T_1 %	T_2 %	T_3 %	T_4 %	Suspected cases	Suspects %	Cases and suspects %
31,878	2,394	55.2	37.3	5.9	1.6	895	2.8	10.3

Source: Pintus, L.; Latte, B., 'Stato Attuale di Diffusione del tracoma', 537

First grade children had a higher index of trachoma than their elders since they had no prior ophthalmic examination. Most municipalities were without nursery schools, so children were visited for the first time only at the age of six and

63 ASNU, EPA, dispensaries, from A to N, 1.15.10, Macomer folder.

showed a higher percentage of T1 and T2, which are the most contagious stages of the disease. Investigations of the homes of the 1,555 trachoma-affected children aged 6-12 years attending summer camps between 1954 and 1959 were not encouraging:

> 'Only few towns in the lowland or in areas favoured by commercial routes have decent and comfortable habitations. The mountain villages have primitive houses built with stones and mud, completely deprived of running water: 80.6% of them do not have any kind of toilet while 19.4% have a rudimentary latrine'.[64]

Nearly three-quarters of the houses had three rooms or less and almost one-half had only two rooms or less. More than 53 per cent of trachoma-affected children lived in houses composed of one or two rooms: worse, the average number of people living in one-room houses was no less than 7.5 and in two-room houses was 4.1.[65] Moreover, the use of such rooms was very general, as places where the entire family and sometimes even animals lived, worked, ate and slept, with sleeping arrangements, summarised in Figure 1.

Fig. 1 Houses of trachoma affected children: bed crowding

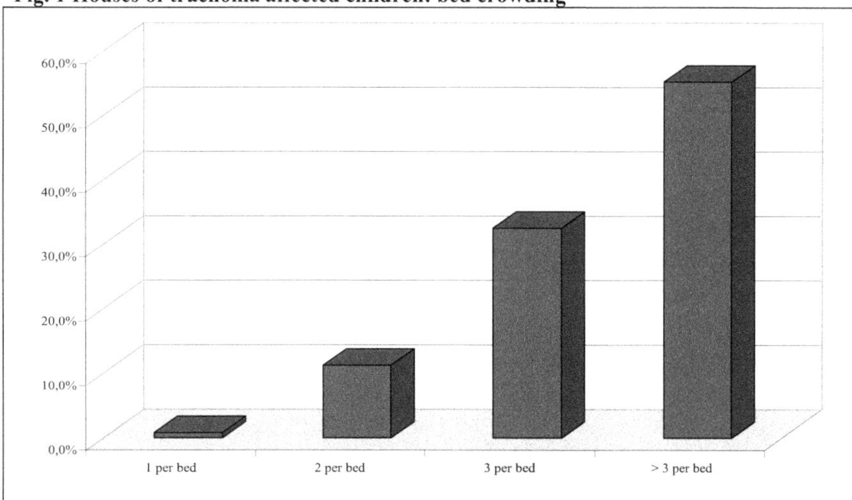

Source: Pintus L., Latte, B., 'Alcuni Aspetti delle Condizioni Igienico-Sanitarie', 711.

64 Pintus, L. and Latte, B. 'Considerazioni sulla Lotta Antitracomatosa....' Nota II'. In *L'Igiene Moderna*, LIII, n. 11-12. 1960, 687-705; Pintus, L. and Latte, B, 'Alcuni Aspetti delle Condizioni Igienico-Sanitarie ed Economico-Sociali dei Tracomatosi in Provincia di Nuoro. Nota III '. In *L'Igiene Moderna*, LIII, n. 11-12. 1960,705-23.

65 Pintus L. and Latte, B., 'Alcuni Aspetti delle Condizioni Igienico-Sanitarie', 707.

Inevitably house size, lack of hygienic services and overcrowding had epidemiological consequences, confirming the statement that the 'crèche is the cradle of trachoma', [66] with a familial trachoma index of 89 per cent, with two or more members of the family being affected by the disease, while only 11 per cent of the contagion was extra-familial. Physical examination of children in summer camps revealed that most were underweight and shorter than average and a study of the diet followed at home, based upon a 60 families sample, is summarised in Table 4.

Table 4 Results of diet survey in summer camps children (Nuoro province 1954-59)

Food type	Amount min. (grams)	Amount max (grams)	Calories min	Calories max
Bread	100	200	361	721
Pasta	40	50	139	174
Cheese	20	40	103	205
Dried legumes	20	30	69	104
Fresh legumes	100	200	39	79
Fats	20	30	164	247
Milk	100	150	67	100
Total			942	1629

Source: Pintus L., Latte, B., 'Alcuni Aspetti delle Condizioni Igienico-Sanitarie', 717.

Even if not accurate for each individual child, these data revealed the poverty and scant nutritional quality of the children's diet in the growing phase of their lives and explained the low body/mass index and signs of rickets observed at the beginning of their stay in the summer camps. After 60 days of better nutrition with 2,500 calories, antibiotic treatment and physical exercises, more than 80 per cent of children were reported to have reached a clinical cicatrisation phase and a better body/mass index.[67]

Trachoma in Talana and Urzulei

Urzulei was selected in 1927 for a new dispensary since five to ten per cent of the local population were affected by trachoma and 25 per cent of school children. Talana meanwhile had only between one and five per cent. [68] The Urzulei

66 Taylor, H., *Trachoma: A Blinding Scourge*, 97.

67 The doctors themselves, pleased by the results obtained in only 60 days, lamented that children would return to their original dismal conditions once discharged by the summer camps and that the Health Ministry would only favour these types of temporary institutions. See Pintus, L. and Latte, B. 'Alcuni Aspetti delle Condizioni Igienico-Sanitarie', 703.

68 See Mura, F. 'Problemi Sociali Isolani: il Tracoma'. In the archives it is much more difficult to find data on Talana than on Urzulei: Talana's Municipal archive has been

general practitioner sent an alarming report to the Nuoro Prefect denouncing the poor health status of the population in his care. He grouped the various diseases into ocular disorders, tubercular forms, malaria and infectious diseases and felt the ocular disorders were the most important and pressing problem, given their 'great diffusion and the serious consequences'.[69] There were at least 50 cases of trachoma and leukoma with total loss of vision in a population of about 1,000 people. The general clinic where he operated had medications to be given only at the time of visit but there were neither pharmacies in the village nor medicines to sustain treatments at home.

In 1933-36 some Urzulei teachers recorded the village doctor's visit, his detection of children affected by trachoma and his order that they visit the local clinic to receive specific cures.[70] This doctor had attended special trachoma courses at the University of Cagliari in 1928, and received a special premium in connection with his anti-trachoma work and for medicines distributed to the general population.[71] The construction of the elementary school building, deliberated upon since 1924, had still not commenced, 'with grave danger to the health of children and teachers for the use of un-hygienic rooms'.[72] Again in 1948, numerous petitions were sent by the Urzulei Mayor and the local doctor to the Prefect and the school superintendent to secure the use of a classroom as village clinic because the small room at the disposal of the doctor was grossly inadequate.[73] The school superintendent was indignant that the Mayor might agree

partially lost and in Nuoro State Archive, the administrative files relative to this village are often empty.

69 ASNU, Fondo Prefettura, EPA dispensaries 1.15.10 (Urzulei folder).

70 Talana and Urzulei contemporary school registers are kept in the Urzulei middle school (ASMU, 'School Registers') but Talana old school records are lost. For Urzulei we consulted the registers from 1920 to 1965. In the 1920s and 1930s, these school registers reveal the terrible conditions of children and classrooms in mountain villages: no school building but dark and dank rooms, with no heating during the extremely cold winter months. The children were barefoot, with ragged and insufficient clothes. They were dirty and uncombed. Both boys and girls were often absent because they were sick or sent to work by the parents.

71 F. Mura (1929) reports the names of all the doctors following the courses on prophylaxis, diagnosis and cure offered in 1927 and 1928 by the Royal Eye Clinic in Cagliari. Only one came from Ogliastra, Dr. Vincenzo Loddo, who was the general practitioner in Urzulei 1933-36. Urzulei Middle School Archive (ASMU) 1930, Urzulei Municipal Archive (ACU) 1934, Mura, 192.

72 ASNU, fondo Prefettura, cat XIII, Gabinetto, folder n. 133.

73 The Urzulei general practitioner, Dr. L. De Nale, wrote to the Mayor 'This narrow and unhygienic ground floor room is rented from a very poor man who occupies the upstairs room with its ten children. During the night apparently the children pee on the floor and the liquid seeps through the ceiling! Moreover there is no waiting area and the sick have to wait in the street their turn to enter. To make matter worse, from the window anybody

that one of the four rooms used for classes in the municipal building might be taken for another purpose.[74] Shortage of space meant that each grade took morning or afternoon sessions only.[75] A second grade teacher coming from the Turin province reported that his students 'do not know the Italian language, cannot read and write and do not know the numbers'.[76] Similarly the fourth and fifth grade teacher found that his classes lacked even rudimentary notions of chemistry and physics: 'in this desolate place, children never saw a car, an electrical lamp, a radio, any type of laboratory!'[77]

In 1951 a new village doctor sent another report to the Urzulei Mayor, lamenting that his previous two reports and requests had gone unattended. In a clinic deprived of any equipment and lacking any pharmaceutical support, attempts to cure patients were a desperate enterprise. He estimated that 25 per cent of the general population was still affected by trachoma but that few sought or could maintain the curative measures required. He reminded the Mayor that trachoma cases were excluded from higher level schools, factory work, military careers and any possibility of emigration. The trachoma clinic was now held in the municipal building, leaving just two classrooms 'where four groups of scholars take turns'.[78] Only in 1960-61 did school registers record the first separate multilevel class for first and second grade trachoma-affected children.[79] From then until 1965, multi-level classes were formed grouping first-second grades and third-fourth-fifth grades. (See Table 5)

---

passing by, can see what is done in the clinic and people are reluctant to come and be cured because of total lack of privacy'. In 1950 we find that Dr. De Nale has been nominated Director of the Urzulei public anti-trachoma surgery (ASNU, Fondo Pref. EPA, Dispensaries 1.15.10, Urzulei folder).

74 He wrote to the Prefect 'the use of a classroom seems neither useful nor rational... It's incredible that a Mayor would be the one to create problems to the School, essential instrument to be protected and cured, ... going against all directives and principles' (ASNU, Fondo Prefettura, EPA Dispensaries 1.15.10, Urzulei folder, 1948).

75 ASNU, fondo Prefettura, EPA, Dispensaries 1.15.10, Urzulei folder.

76 ASMU 1949-50, School registers

77 ASMU, 1946-47, School registers

78 ACU, Sanità, 1951, letter of Dr. Alfieri Pozzar to the Mayor. He also reminded the Mayor that the village hygienic conditions were appalling since there was no sewage system and the cemetery was completely inadequate.

79 ASMU, 1960-61, School registers

Table 5 Enrolled and trachoma affected children in Urzulei elementary school (1961-65)

School year	Total number of children	Trachoma affected children	Trachoma affected %
1961-62	174	40	23.0
1962-63	203	35	17.2
1963-64	208	25	12.0
1964-65	214	14	6.5

Source: ASMU, School registers

Urzulei data show that, in the early 1960s, the percentage of trachoma-affected children in Sardinia was still almost the double of that in southern Italy and in Sicily.[80] The 1960s marked a period of economic boom for Italy that changed the social conditions of the population. In Talana and Urzulei, antibiotic drugs finally became available but another drastic change was caused by emigration, as remittances allowed the possibility of building new houses with the modern comforts of tiled floors, running water, indoor toilets and electricity. These offered the means of attaining cleanliness without having to walk several miles to the water fountains.

As seen in the city of Sassari and in the town of Alghero the fight against trachoma began early in the twentieth century with many sanitary initiatives and by the 1940s sulpha drugs therapy had been introduced in all the provincial centres. Yet even with a progressive decrease in the prevalence of the disease and a reduction of its most serious complications, the complete eradication of trachoma was attained only after significant improvements in hygienic infrastructures, notably the availability and treatment of drinking water and better housing and amenities. The medical solution is important but not sufficient without corresponding improvement in the hygienic conditions of the communities. This is clearly demonstrated by the enduring presence of trachoma in third world countries where millions of dollars are spent on the distribution of medication but insufficient effort is employed, even today, to ensure that people have the ready and easy availability of water for personal hygiene. As Ida Mann, a British ophthalmologist visiting the Australian outback and treating many Aboriginal people with trachoma, said in 1966 'Drugs? I'd prescribe water. If governments were to put water on, nobody would have trachoma!'[81] Doctors and ophthalmologists engaged in the trachoma battle in Sardinia were well aware of this more than fifty years earlier, as demonstrated by Sotgia in 1913:

---

80 Luzzo, S. *Salute e sanità nell'Italia repubblicana, Rome*, Donzelli, 2004, 390.

81 Mann, I. *Culture, Race, Climate and Eye Disease*, Springfield, Illinois, Charles C. Thomas, 1966, quoted in Taylor, *Trachoma: A Blinding Scourge*, 175.

'Trachoma will continue to populate our streets with blind people, force valid youths branded by disablement into idleness and dependency on domestic and municipal support, if we do not understand that trachoma is the disease of illiteracy and of filth that can be won over only with schooling and abundant water for attaining cleanliness in the person and in the home.'[82]

82 Sotgia, G. M. *Il tracoma nelle scuole elementari di Sassari*, 11-12.

THE PUBLIC HEALTH ROLE OF RURAL MEDICAL PRACTITIONERS: NORFOLK AND FIFE C. 1860-1914

Steven Cherry

In 1881 the critic Frances Power Cobbe wrote in the *Modern Review* that, 'As medical officers in parishes and (poor law) unions, factory and prison surgeons, public vaccinators, medical officers of health, inspectors of nuisances and very commonly as coroners, the doctors are daily assuming authority.'[1] Whilst deploring this trend, she nevertheless summarised the expanding public role of medical practitioners, linked by some contemporaries to a growing medicalisation of everyday life.[2] The rural dimensions of this change, and of the doctors' role, have recently been re-examined and this essay takes up a related but neglected aspect, the early public health work of general medical practitioners in the countryside.[3] Case examples from Norfolk (eastern England) and Fife (east-central Scotland) are used as the basis for more provisional generalisations, once the emerging structures of rural public health have been outlined.

Reform of the English poor laws in 1834 created some 600 Unions or administrative areas, each run by locally elected Boards of Guardians under limited central supervision. Stigmatised relief to able bodied paupers was meant to be confined within a system of workhouses, but the destitute received indoor or outdoor assistance and limited medical provision was made for the sick and infirm. Under the General Medical Orders of 1842 medical sub-districts of up to 15,000 acres or 15,000 people began to be established within each poor law union, under the responsibility of qualified District Medical Officers (DMOs), 'duly licensed to practice as medical men.'[4] Although the initial focus was upon

---

1 Cobbe, F.P. 'The medical profession and its morality', *The Modern Review*, 2, (1881), 296-328, 297.

2 For a fierce critique see Shaw, G.B. 'Preface on Doctors', in *The Doctor's Dilemma* (1906), Penguin Harmondsworth, 1982, 9-88.

3 Cherry, S.'Medicine and Rural Health Care in 19th Century Europe' and 'General practitioners, Hospitals and Medical Services in England: the East Anglia Region 1800-1948', in Barona, J.L and Cherry, S. *Health and Medicine in Rural Europe*, Valencia, PUV, Seminari d'Estudis sobre la Ciencia, 2005, 19-62 and 171-191.

4 Hodgkinson, R.G. *The Origins of the National Health Service: the medical services of the new Poor Law 1834-1871*, London, Wellcome Historical Library, 1967, 14-15, 23; Muncaster, M. J. 'Medical Services and the Medical Profession in Norfolk 1815-1911', unpublished PhD thesis, Norwich, UEA, 1976. These limits were meant to avoid exploitation of doctors, although remuneration was left to the guardians and questions involving travel and process, notably the role of poor law relieving officers in medical care, were not resolved.

sick paupers, these sub-districts later became part of the structure of rural public health. Sanitary legislation in 1866 required the appointment of urban officials – principally a qualified Medical Officer of Health (MoH) and usually one or more sanitary inspectors in an assisting role. Corresponding officials were added in rural areas in 1872 after poor law and public health measures were combined under the Local Government Board in 1871. But whereas distinct urban sanitary authorities were established from 1872, the existing poor law Boards of Guardians took on this role in the countryside, the respective authorities renamed as Urban and Rural District Councils (UDCs, RDCs) following the 1888 Local Government Act. Although actual provisions varied considerably, rural areas thus developed a governmental structure comprised of local parish, district and county councils.

Scotland had a separate poor law and, between the 1845 Poor Law Act and the 1892 Local Government Act, this saw the more limited grouping of parishes under the London-based Board of Supervision. Many parishes, particularly those in rural areas under the influence of local landowners, combined harsh attitudes towards the poor with flexibility in provision, for example offering limited forms of outdoor relief or using local charitable effort. Although medical relief for the sick, disabled or infirm was encouraged by government grants from 1848, the grassroots delivery of services was haphazard. For example, local voluntary hospitals might be utilised where these existed and poorhouses accommodated the destitute, aged and children as well as the chronic sick, but even this mixed accommodation, let alone the facilities of a hospital ward, was rare outside the larger towns. [5]

This did not augur well for public health provision. Following the 1862 Burgh Police and Improvement Act, Scotland's 1867 Public Health Act charged the Board of Supervision with disease control, the removal of nuisances and regulation of lodging houses, and it also enabled parochial boards in rural areas to appoint MosH and sanitary inspectors. [6] Yet the Board had limited powers and there was no guarantee that medical officers would undertake or be paid for public health work, particularly in more remote or rural areas where sanitary inspectors were very much part-time officials. [7] Some 34 county councils were

---

5 Levitt, I. *Poverty and Welfare in Scotland 1890-1948*, Edinburgh, Edinburgh University Press, 1988, 12.

6 'Circular as to bye-laws for Sanitary Inspectors', 28 March 1873, *Board of Supervision (BoS) Annual Report 1873*, Vol. XXXV1,1874, Appendix A, No.17, 46-47, in Levitt, I. (ed.) *Government and Social Conditions in Scotland 1845-1919*, Edinburgh, Scottish History Society, 1988, 13. Public hospital provision was also encouraged but Scotland had less than 1,500 beds for the infectious sick in 1890.

7 For example, a Board circular to medical officers in 1869 urged them *not* to undertake health surveys etc 'as would seriously interfere with your ordinary duties as General Superintendents of Poor. They might enquire 'how far the enactments of the Public Health

established under the 1889 Local Government (Scotland) Act and, from 1892, the Local Government Board replaced the Board of Supervision. With one full-time medical official within the executive assisting the Scottish Secretary, the possibilities of greater technical input on public health matters improved. Further, one hundred or so larger villages were added to the existing burghs responsible as district councils for providing water, drainage and scavenging services. This complex of arrangements offered no guarantee of effectiveness, however. As seen above, medical officers had no positive indications as to any wider perception of their public health duties and the rural districts tended to lack the resources to support the doctors' efforts: 'with the majority having a population of less than 5,000, they had neither the finance, nor the work, for a full-time public health department … to ensure they successfully implemented the public health and housing laws. The evidence suggests … a particularly uphill struggle.' [8]

Norfolk was divided into ten urban and twenty rural sanitary districts, the latter with a combined 1881 census population of 266,400 at a low density averaging one person per 4.66 acres. The county appeared to epitomise 'the healthy rural' since, omitting the main population centres of Norwich, Yarmouth and Kings Lynn, its crude death rates varied between nine and seventeen per cent below national averages. Given the higher age distribution of this rural population, standardised death rates were still lower, as was the incidence of principal diseases such as tuberculosis, typhoid, measles, and scarlet fever. Similarly with infant diahorreal deaths, although an early fall in infant mortality rates, from 164 to 131 per 1,000 births between 1851-1881, was not sustained.[9] One local study has already considered the possibility that 'quite a lot of people in rural Norfolk stood to benefit, at least on the margin, from the measures of rural district councils by the early twentieth century'.[10]

---

are complied with, and ….you will report the same (failures) to the Board' which did 'not expect' full or rapid implementation of the 1867 Act. *BoS Annual Report 1869*, vol XXXV, 1870 Appendix A, No 9. In: Levitt, *Social Conditions in Scotland*, 11-12.

8 Levitt (ed.) *Social Conditions in Scotland*, Introduction xx; Levitt, *Poverty and Welfare in Scotland*, 24.

9 Excluding Norwich, Kings Lynn and Great Yarmouth, the rural Norfolk quinquennial CDR fell from 17.6/1,000 1876-80 to 17.1 1886-90, 15.7 1896-1900 and 13.4 1906-10. Armstrong, A. *The Population of Victorian and Edwardian Norfolk*, Norwich, Centre of East Anglian Studies, 2000, 49-53.

10 Armstrong, *The Population of Victorian and Edwardian Norfolk*, 67. The rural Norfolk CDR 1906-10 was 13.4, compared with 14.2 for all Norfolk and 14.7 for England and Wales. The rural Norfolk IMR was also less, though with no pronounced fall before the early 1900s (viz. late 1896-1900 143 and 1906-10 103). This 'sticky' IMR kept up the late 19th century CDR, with the greatest saving of lives (comparing the 1900-2 mortality with that for 1870-2) occurring among adults (aged 15+ , 45 %), children and older children (4-14, about 15 %); and then infants (24 %).

Map 1. Norfolk poor law unions 1834 – 1930[11]

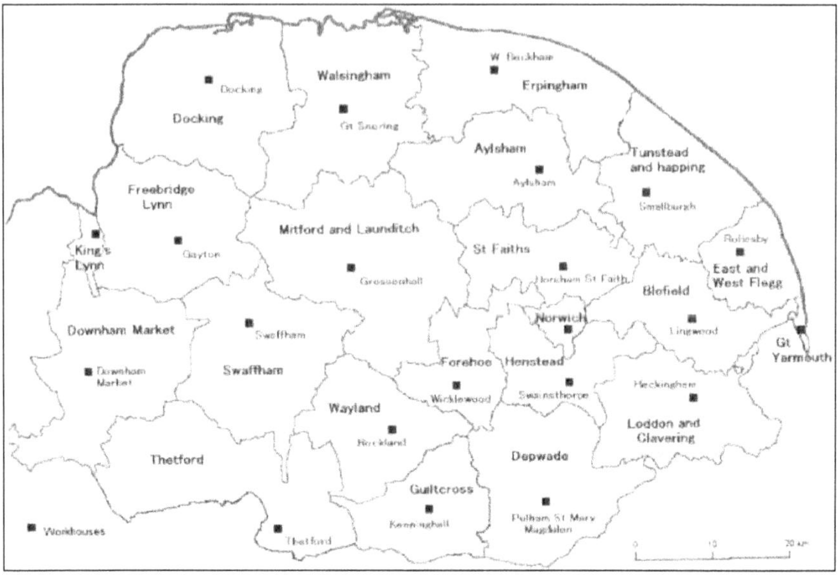

The variability of nineteenth-century health provision suggests caution but, given the limited evidence of better living standards, nutrition or housing improvement in rural areas, it is possible that medical coverage in the countryside, both in terms of doctoring and public health work, has been understated. Roughly two-thirds of Norfolk doctors worked as part-time DMOs, typically in areas of about 20 square miles.[12] Most were assisted by sanitary inspectors and, given Hamilton's suggestion that larger towns rapidly developed standardised public health procedures from the 1870s, a study of these rural agencies of public health, using RDC sanitary committees and MosH records, seems worthwhile. [13]

Whatever the claims of the 'healthy rural', Norfolk MosH frequently reported on defective housing, water supplies and sanitation and also alleged

11 From Ashwin, T. and Davison, A. *An Historical Atlas of Norfolk*, Chichester, Phillimore, 2005, Map 71, 148.

12 Digby, A. *Pauper Palaces*, London, Routledge and Keegan Paul, 1978, 166-7. For example, the Smallburgh (NE Norfolk) RDC area in 1901 had 17,000+ population and four medical districts, with each DMO paid £78 per annum. Report by Dr McVail on Smallburgh Union, Norfolk. In: *Report of the Royal Commission on the Poor Laws and Relief of Distress*, London, HMSO, 1909. XIV, 180-2.

13 Hamilton, C. 'Sanitary policing and the local state', *Social History of Medicine*. 18, (2005), 39-61, 55-6.

parental negligence, variously citing the reluctance to have children vaccinated; insufficient provision for medical attendance; drinking from contaminated ponds or wells; and resort to opium to relieve marsh fever in low-lying areas. [14] Their early investigations were frequently moralistic and judgemental. For example, an 1863 study of excessive mortality of infants in English rural districts noted that three of the five areas selected were in Norfolk. Environmental features such as a low-lying location were seen as background contributors, though drainage improvements were also acknowledged, as was the switch to arable farming and its associated greater female employment, especially in the gang labour system, which was singled out as a particular problem. Gang women were allegedly 'tainted with a customary immorality', reflected in illegitimacies, premature births, neglect of their babies, use of opium and prevalence of diahorrea and fevers. Indeed, the prevailing but unsympathetic opinion of poor law DMOs at the time concerning infant mortality was said to be 'that under whatever late symptoms the death was recorded, the real cause of half of them was the mother's neglect. The degree of criminality attributed to the women varied, from a sympathizing excuse for their ignorance to … willful neglect with the hope of death, - in fact infanticide.' [15]

A different approach, based upon information provided by local MosH and sanitary inspectors, was reflected in the first Norfolk County MoH report, issued in 1889. Dr Shepard Taylor noted more than 350 nuisances from closets, over 160 instances of defective drainage and at least 90 of defective water supplies, with a dozen or so cases each involving refuse, manure heaps, animals, overcrowding, dilapidated housing, filthy premises, and slaughter houses. This snapshot of county-wide health investigation that year also included a glimpse of practical improvements undertaken, including nearly 50 new or repaired closets, over 100 new water closets or conversions; and almost 70 new, repaired or

14 Across Europe similar remarks were made concerning the rural poor at this time. English sanitary legislation stated that 'Any dwellings which owing to dampness, defective ventilation, or other causes, are in the opinion of the MoH unfit for human habitation, should at once be put in proper repair or permanently closed'. MosH acquired similar powers to deal with 'nuisances'; after the notification of infectious disease (particularly after 1890 Act), with disinfection etc. Their responsibilities later extended to isolation hospitals; antitoxin v. diphtheria; diagnosis in 'doubtful', 'contact' or 'overlooked' TB cases; provision of advice or training (eg TB cases, childbirth); and nursing care for the home treatment of puerperal fever. LGB Memorandum 'On unification of official medical services for the poor', cited in 1909 *Royal Commission on the Poor Laws*, Majority Report, Part V Medical Relief, 303-85, 337.

15 Hunter, H.J. 'Report on the excessive mortality of infants in some rural districts of England', Appendix 14 to *Sixth Report of the Medical Officer of the Privy Council 1863*, (1864) 454-462, 456-7. The Norfolk areas cited were west (Freebridge Lynn) and east (Great Yarmouth) coastal districts and the Wayland /Buckenham/ Guiltcross area, south west of Norwich.

cleaned wells and other well closures. There were also sixteen school closures to contain infectious outbreaks, with indications that more were to be expected once the 1890 Infectious Disease (Notification) Act came into force and MosH could begin to exercise their powers in response to official alerts of outbreak or 'nuisance.'[16]

Scotland's crude death rates (CDR) averaged 22 per 1,000 in 1860s and 1870s, falling particularly in the 1890s and early 1900s and thereafter at a decelerating rate.[17] Flinn's compilation for rural Scotland suggested a lower CDR initially, perhaps 17-18 per 1,000 1861-91, and from these differentials he concluded that defective sanitary conditions in towns and cities were so bad 'that urbanisation rather than poverty was the cause of high mortality in the mid nineteenth century.' [18] Nevertheless there was subsequently less evidence of continuing improvement in rural areas and, although tuberculosis, fevers and whooping cough were most destructive in the towns, outbreaks of diphtheria, typhoid and influenza and some mortality variations suggest that a healthy environment or effective medical services could not be assumed in the countryside.[19] Although rural depopulation may have produced an ageing demographic structure, with proportionately fewer deaths from childhood infectious diseases, a few hitherto rural or coastal areas saw significant industrial and population growth.

Fife was a good example of such change, as its population increased rapidly from 154,000 inhabitants in 1851 to 267,700 by 1911. This growth was associated with an upsurge in the mining and exporting of coal from the middle of the nineteenth century, which stimulated other industrial activity and offset the lack of development in the older linen trades and fishing. St Andrews was the old university town but Cowdenbeath and Dunfirmline expanded rapidly, respecttively as coalmining and ironfounding centres, while Kirkaldy, Methil and Buckhaven (formerly a major fishing centre) grew as a result of coal exports. County crude death rates declined from averages of roughly 19 per 1,000 1860-75, to 17 or so 1875-90 and to 15 1901-5; somewhere between Scotland's

16 Norfolk Record Office (NRO) C/MH 1/1 *Norfolk Medical Officer of Heath Report 1889* (Shepard T. Taylor), 23; and see footnote 14 above.

17 viz. 20.5 in 1880; 18.5 1900; 15.3 1910; 14,0 1920; 13.3 1930 and 13.2 1945. Mitchell, B.R. (ed.) *International Historical Statistics; Europe 1750-1988*, London, Macmillan, 1992, entries for Scotland, 99, 106, 118, 120.

18 viz. 16.6 in 1901; 14.2 1911; 13.0 1921 and 12.8 1931. Flinn, M.W. et al, *Scottish Population History*, Cambridge, Cambridge University Press, 1977, 382.

19 Flinn, *Scottish Population History*, 389. Kinross, adjoining Fife, had a small, sparse and fluctuating population of 8,900 in 1851 but just 6,700 1891, partly recovering to 7,500 in 1911. It had a similarly fluctuating and much less obvious mortality decline: CDR 16.1 1855-60 and still 15.2 1936-9, with peak mortality of 20.8 in the late 1870s. ibid, 380-1.

national and 'rural' averages, but these also tended to decelerate during the interwar years.20

Map 2. East/Central Scotland

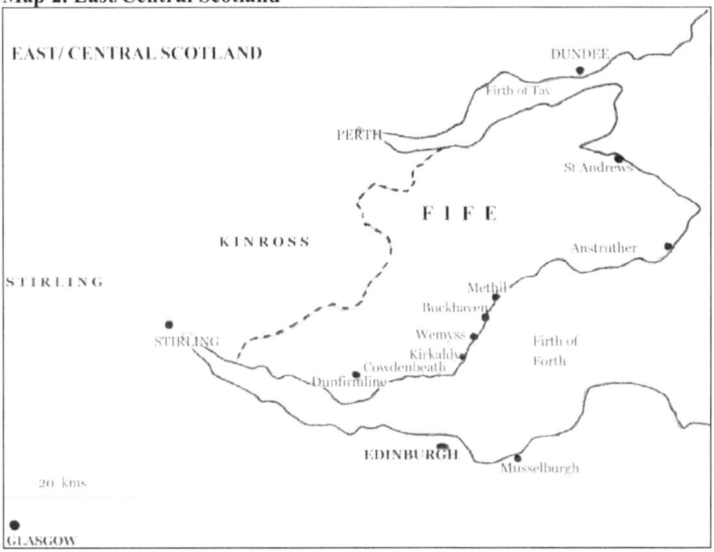

The Board of Supervision's part-time medical officer, Dr Littlejohn, visited Fife on several occasions and painted a depressing picture of public health arrangements in Scottish rural areas generally before 1900. Following a typhoid outbreak outside Glasgow in 1875, which was traced to farm-contaminated milk in the county of Renfrew, he noted that local parish doctors

> 'have not been appointed Officers of Health … under the Public Health (Scotland) Act … and are not called upon to take any sanitary supervision of the villages in the parish. The Sanitary Inspector is also the Poor Law Officer, and has the supervision of a very large parish, and the salary he receives for sanitary work is nearly nominal … (and) with the arrangements common to Scotch villagers, of (concerning) middens, wells, and water courses, disease germinates freely in all directions.' [21]

Possibly this depiction was too generalised or pessimistic, but it applied to many parts of rural Scotland. More than a century later, Ian Levitt's study of the Board

---

20 viz. CDR 14.1 1911-15; 12.1 1921-5 and still 12.1 1936-9.

21 'Report on Typhoid fever at Crosshill, Parish of Cathcart', Dr Littlejohn, 28 April 1875, *BoS Annual Report 1874-5*, XXXII 1875, App A, No. 14, 128-35, in Levitt (ed.) *Social Conditions in Scotland*, 128.

of Supervision has also noted its preoccupation with urban-industrial Scotland, rather than the Highlands or the rural south. Perhaps more surprisingly, his interpretation of Scottish medical officers' evidence to the Royal Commission on the Poor Law (Vol XLVI) in 1910 was that 'they were so overwhelmed by Poor Law matters that their inspections under the Public Health Act declined.' [22]

Such conclusions might be compared with Crowther's summation that medical reform impulses within the English Poor Law also weakened after the 1860s. [23] As both views indicate the danger of simply assuming rural health improvements by the early twentieth century, the next section considers examples of public health effort, focusing upon defective housing; water supplies and drainage; and isolation measures, in the context of the realities of rural life.

The Healthy Rural?

To begin with housing, Norfolk had many landed estates but rather fewer 'model' landowners willing to use their wealth to enhance housing and other amenities offered to their tenants and employees. A particular problem was that large landowners were able to restrict labour and housing in 'close' parishes under their control so that, in remaining 'open' parishes, there was a grim combination of casual or underemployed labour on low wages with speculative building and overcrowding, as tenants looked to subdivide rents. Dr H. J. Hunter's *Report on the Rural labourers' housing* to the Privy Council in 1864 noted how some landlords combined self-interest and Malthusian perspectives: they 'look on the people as a surging fluid anxious to find its own level and ruinous wherever it comes. To give it vent will be to render their beloved estate uninhabitable and to eat it up with poor rates.'[24] Evictions from 'close' parishes caused labourers to travel great distances to get work and to crowd into available housing, described as 'small and dear, crammed with grown up children and lodgers.'[25] He also cited examples of unsympathetic and judgemental opinion on people in these 'open' parishes: 'the scum of the neighbourhood settles down on this spot:

---

22 Levitt (ed.) *Social Conditions in Scotland*, Introduction, xiv, xvii.

23 Crowther, M.A. 'Paupers or patients? Obstacles to Professionalisation in the Poor Law Medical Service before 1914', *Journal History of Medicine*, 39, (1984), 33-54, 34.

24 Hunter, H.J. 'Inquiry on the State of the Dwellings of Rural Labourers', Appendix 6, *Seventh Report of the Medical Officer of the Privy Council* (1864), London, HMSO, 1865, 126-303, 235.

25 Similarly 'people roaming by day over miles of depopulated country… clustering and wrangling for lodgings at night like rats on the mast of a sinking ship'. Appendix 6, *Seventh Report of the Medical Officer of the Privy Council* (1864), London, HMSO, 1865, 234-5.

for should a man lose his honesty or a woman her virtue, both are ejected from the close parish and of course take up their abode in the next open one.'[26]

Although people as much as the environment might be problematised, some rural housing seemed to be designed as slums, without proper foundations, floors or drainage, compounded by defective roofing and the lack of gutters, which made walls damp.[27] Local authorities initially had few powers or the inclination to act: thus in East Norfolk, again in 1864, 'Mr Burroughes, proprietor of a considerable estate, was summoned before the magistrates on the ground that some of his cottages at Hamblingdon and South Walsham were ... legal nuisances, and although the facts were proved, the only part of the charge on which he could be convicted proved to be the omission to provide privies.'[28] A related rural housing feature was the 'one up, one down' combination of a bedroom over a combined kitchen and living room. In the village of Denver, West Norfolk, 20 of the 24 cottages inspected in 1864 had just one bedroom each and these accommodated in total 62 adults and 69 children.[29] Such conditions were tolerated in the absence of cheap or alternative provision and, as the Aylsham MoH was still reporting in 1911, 'the occupiers ... especially in those parishes where cottages are scarce, are generally disinclined to make complaints, and are content to live under conditions prejudicial to health.'[30]

Particularly in the more remote rural areas, the mere monitoring of health nuisances, let alone their remedy, posed major problems. As one Scottish official complained, 'anything approaching to a complete inspection of the large extent of country in my district is impossible. I am under the necessity of taking much on trust from reports of the local Sanitary Inspectors ... (which) ... to a large extent are merely nominal.'[31] Such circumstances might give rise to

---

26 (Read) 'Report on Norfolk Farming', *Journal of the Royal Agricultural Society*, Vol. XIX, 293, cited Appendix 6, *Seventh Report of the Medical Officer of the Privy Council* (1864), London, HMSO, 1865, 234.

27 Linsley, B. 'Homes for Heroes. Housing legislation and its effect on housing in rural Norfolk 1918-39', unpublished PhD thesis, UEA, 2005. She cites A. Wilson Fox's depiction of a rural slum, in Gaskell, M.S. (ed) *Slums*, London, Leicester University Press, 1990, 126: 'overcrowding in the sleeping rooms, low ceilings, small windows, rickety stairs, while downstairs the living room is often a small kitchen possessing no back door, where the cooking and washing have to be done. The discomfort of illness in such places can be imagined. Add to this, dampness on the ground floor, general want of repair, little or no garden, no proper outhouse or sanitary arrangements, and water to be fetched from some distance, and occasionally nothing but pondwater to be obtained...'

28 Hunter, 'Dwellings of Rural Labourers', 235.

29 Hunter, 'Dwellings of Rural Labourers', 235-6.

30 NRO, C/MH1/7b, Aylsham, 99.

31 A. Campbell, Inspecting Officer for Highlands (Southern) District, *BoS Annual Report 1883-4*, Vol. XXXVIII 1884, App. A, No. 6, 19. In Levitt (ed.) *Social Conditions in Scotland*, 16.

generalisations from certain extreme cases, but the deficiencies in much of Scottish housing accommodation were obvious and few remedies were found. Even in 1917, the Royal Commission on Housing in Scotland reported not just on urban slums but on general crowding, lack of water supplies, refuse disposal and basic amenities, along with 'the persistence of the unspeakably filthy privy-midden in many of the mining areas; badly constructed, incurably damp labourers cottages on farms; whole townships unfit for human occupation in the crofting counties and islands …' [32] This does not suggest wholesale later nineteenth-century improvements but crude indicators, such as the average number of persons per inhabited house, suggest appreciably greater problems in Scotland, with roughly eight persons per habitation 1851-1881, compared with between five and six in England and Wales. [33]

If Glasgow's slum tenements achieved especial notoriety, Scotland's housing problems were geographically diverse and took specific forms. For example, many rural areas had communal 'bothy' accommodation: barrack-like and usually for male farm labourers, this was a far cry from the idealised rural family cottage, though at least it represented provision usually separated from animal livestock. [34] With industrial growth in new areas these arrangements were increasingly extended to temporary workers; for example, to women employed in dyeing and bleaching textiles. In mining areas such as Fife much of the colliery housing was tied in to the work, which meant that tenants had neither security in employment nor accommodation and houses were often shoddily built, lacking in amenities and poorly maintained. More generally, land sales in Scotland involved the payment of an annual duty to former vendors, the 'feu-duty', which pushed up land values and encouraged land hoarding in anticipation of still higher prices. As a result, those able to secure land for house-building paid dearly and therefore looked to provide high-density accommodation. But with average wages in Scottish industrialising areas reckoned at between ten and twenty per cent less than in England, subdivision and overcrowding was almost guaranteed, as was the threat to the inhabitants' health. [35] Thus in Fife, more than 67 per cent of the Cowdenbeath population lived two per room – and 37 per

---

32 *Report of the Royal Commission on the Housing of the Induistrial Population of Scotland Rural and Urban* London, HMSO, 1917, para 2232. In Cramond, R.D. *Housing Policy in Sotland 1919-1964*, Edinburgh, Oliver and Boyd, 1964, 80.

33 Gauldie, E. *Cruel Habitations: a history of working class housing 1780-1918*, London, Allen and Unwin, 1973, Appendix 2, 319.

34 Gauldie, *Cruel Habitations*, 66-7.

35 Rodger, R. 'Crisis and confrontation in Scottish housing 1880-1914', in Rodger, R. (ed.) *Scottish Housing in the Twentieth Century*, Leicester, Leicester University Press, 1989, 25-53, 25-6.

cent lived three per room – in 1911, and similarly almost 50 per cent in Kirkaldy and nearly 40 per cent in Dunfirmline.[36]

A related problem concerned drainage and water supplies. Although population density in Norfolk was low, the heavy reliance upon wells and ponds exposed people to water pollution. Early health intervention successes in the county included the systematic testing of wells in Walsingham and in Swaffham in 1888, although inadequate responses were being reported in Depwade some two years after initial alerts by the local inspector. [37] The Mitford and Launditch (Mid Norfolk) MoH claimed in 1890 that, over the previous fifteen years, 120 new deep wells were sunk, with 66 others deepened, cleaned or repaired. [38] This represented earlier and supporting evidence for Armstrong's Smallburgh survey (1907-12), where more than 120 wells were cleaned, repaired, or replaced and over 250 'stinking old middens' were superseded by 'dry pail' systems burying excrement away from water courses, arrangements which affected at least one-half of the district population. [39] In contrast Stalham's sanitary inspector surveyed all 256 dwellings in the village in 1912, finding more than 100 with no drains whatsoever so that 'the contents from closets, house refuse, slops and dirty water are all disposed of onto small garden plots … drinking water wells are situated on the same plots.' [40] These very different findings reflected not only variations in local sanitary conditions but also how the latter were problematised by rural health officials.

Fife's more diversified environment featured examples of industrial and rural squalor and some familiar problems. An outbreak of cholera in the coastal town of Wemyss in 1866 peaked with 21 deaths from November 19th-22nd. Dr Littlejohn remarked upon local inactivity and demoralisation but he made arrangements for fumigation and disinfection, the burning of bedding and use of local school rooms to separate the sick who were able to move. He could not but notice defective sanitary arrangements in neighbouring areas: those in the crowded mining village of Methil were 'in a fearful state, with mountains of ash heaps', and in the fishing village of Buckhaven, cramped and hemmed in on a steep incline, middens and fish offal, compounded by pig-keeping, had contaminated

---

36 Rodger, R. 'Crisis and confrontation', 28.

37 NRO C/MH1/2 NCC *Report on the Sanitary Condition of the Administrative County of Norfolk 1894* (H Cooper Pattin), respectively 56, 62, 50.

38 NRO C/MH1/1, *Norfolk MoH Report 1889*, 70-1. The wells were between 7 and 30 metres deep.

39 NRO C/MH1/1, *Norfolk MoH Report 1889*, 39. Armstrong, Population of Norfolk, 49-53.

40 NRO, DC 22/3/30, Stalham RDC, Inspector 1912. Two thirds of houses relied on earth pails but there were still 80 middens, at least one-quarter of which were 'insanitary'.

local wells. He concluded, 'one is tempted to marvel, not that cholera infects such a place (but) that the disease is ever absent.'[41]

Given such infectious disease outbreaks, the provision of isolation facilities was essential. Norfolk's voluntary hospitals were traditionally reluctant to admit the infectious sick so the county relied on its workhouses, most of which offered a partly-isolated 'pest house'. Isolation came to be recognised as both a public and a personal service, yet its continuing association with the poor law in rural areas meant that facilities remained basic and stigmatised. [42] Even with improved understanding of the process of infection, practical arrangements remained limited: in 1896 just eight of Norfolk's 21 poor law unions offered separate infirmaries or infectious wards.[43] Ignorance and authority could also be powerful restraints, with the Earl of Kimberley, chairman of the Forehoe Guardians in 1890s, able to prevent even the installation of baths at the Wicklewood workhouse because he considered bathing a danger to health.[44] So although the 1866 Sanitary Act encouraged provision and the 1867 Metropolitan Poor Act raised the possibility that poor law facilities might develop into 'state hospitals into which all the sick poor of the country might be received for medical treatment and care', the 1909 Poor Law Minority Report was still urging positive responses in 'many other unions – rural as well as urban.' [45]

Early nineteenth-century Scottish isolation measures relied on the voluntary hospitals, which helped only tiny numbers and has caused some historians to wonder whether such hospitals were as yet medical institutions in the modern sense.[46] Public arrangements could be primitive: the first victim of a fever outbreak in Ardrossan in 1847 was taken to a wooden shed actually located in the town graveyard. This 'temporary fever hospital' had room for one person but lacked even a bed, let alone washing, night visit or attendance facilities, so the already delirious man was laid on boards with bedding, where he remained until he died. [47] Without effective powers the Board of Supervision merely expressed

---

41 Report by Dr H.D. Littlejohn on the Sanitary State of the Parish of Wemyss, 6 December 1866, in *BoS Annual Report 1867* Vol XXXIII (1867-8), App. A, No.11, 17-21, in Levitt (ed.) *Social Conditions in Scotland*, 115-118. This was hardly novel: ineffective, haphazard responses and lack of control over public nuisances had already been emphasised during the 1830-1 and 1848 cholera outbreaks.

42 For discussion of issues surrounding isolation, see Pickstone, J.V. *Medicine and Industrial Society*, Manchester, Manchester University Press, 1985, 181.

43 Digby, *Pauper Palaces*, 169.

44 Digby, *Pauper Palaces*, 169.

45 *20th Annual Report of the Poor Law Board, 1867-8*, 28 cited in *Royal Commission on the Poor Laws and Relief of Distress*, London, HMSO, 1909, 310.

46 Levitt, *Poverty and Welfare in Scotland*, 12.

47 BoS Public Health Minutes, 17 February 1848, Scottish Record Office (SRO), HH23/2, in Levitt, (ed.) *Social Conditions in Scotland*, 114.

hopes that, in general, rural isolation facilities might be provided in vacant cottages or by arrangement with 'trustworthy cottagers not having children, to receive and nurse … patients requiring such accommodation.'[48] Yet the absence of isolation arrangements remained a major defect in many areas. Thus the 1885 typhoid outbreak in Craig, Forfarshire (pop 2,589 in 1881) struck 478 people and led to 40 deaths, 'which in all probability would have been avoided had the local authority been in a position to isolate the first few cases.' Simultaneously, typhoid deaths in Middlebie, Dumfriesshire (pop 1,972 in 1881) were aggravated because the parish 'has no means of isolating cases of infectious disease.' [49]

When local landowners refused even to sell land on which to establish fever hospitals, as in Musselburgh in the early 1870s, the Board urged the authorities to use their statutory powers or railed at their 'dereliction of duty … which will be condemned by the majority of inhabitants and be a source of deep regret to the Local Authority themselves', but was itself powerless. [50] And some local authorities were wilfully ignorant: when those at Wemyss declared it 'inexpedient' to close the local school during a scarletina outbreak in 1874, despite the advice of two parish medical officers, the Board could do no more than condemn their stance as 'far from creditable to the majority either as regards their humanity or their intelligence.'[51]

Shaping rural public health medicine

Conventionally, the later nineteenth century is associated with changes in public health involving preventive medicine; bacteriology; concepts of specificity in disease and a practical focus upon disease notification, isolation and disinfection; as well as the targeting of groups at risk, such as schoolchildren, for various hygiene and disease 'campaigns'.[52] Yet the application of change involved local contexts and interactions, as confirmed by the case studies here.

Most obviously, local authorities might restrict medical effort. The extension of the franchise in 1885 to cover more male householders in the countryside had only limited impact upon landowner authority or representation in national or

---

48 *BoS Annual Report 1872*, Circular 681, Vol XXIX (1873), App A, No.18, 101-3, in Levitt, (ed.) *Social Conditions in Scotland*, 120.

49 Examples cited in BoS Public Health Minutes, 18 November 1886, SRO HH 25/10, in Levitt, (ed.) *Social Conditions in Scotland*, 138.

50 BoS Public Health Minutes, 18 June 1874, SRO, HH 25/4, in Levitt, (ed.) *Social Conditions in Scotland*, 123.

51 BoS Public Health Minutes, 24 December 1874, SRO, HH 25/4, in Levitt, (ed.) *Social Conditions in Scotland*, 124.

52 see Cherry, 'Medicine and Rural Health Care', 40; Fee, E. and Porter, D. 'Public health, preventive medicine and professionalisation: England and America in the nineteenth century'. In Wear, A. (ed) *Medicine and Society*, Cambridge, Cambridge University Press, 1992, 265-75, 270.

local politics initially, and the rural guardians or district sanitary committees continued to reflect farming interests, which were always more likely to see public health in terms of costs rather than value.[53] For example, the Board of Supervision had continuously criticised the authorities in Kirkaldy for two decades because they refused to establish an isolation hospital. In 1896 over 320 reported cases of typhoid and scarlet fever in the district resulted in 30 deaths, including local medical officer Dr Morrison. A subsequent investigation pinpointed the failure to isolate early cases, with 'the negligence of the Kirkaldy authorities to provide suitable hospital accommodation ... typical of some at least among the small Scotch burghs.'[54]

Similarly Anne Digby's pioneering study of Norfolk poor law arrangements suggested that 'the chief impediments to medical progress in rural unions were the prejudices, parsimony and ignorance of the boards of guardians', a view likely to be relevant also to public health.[55] In regard to preventive measures, it was reckoned that almost 70 per cent of English infants were vaccinated against smallpox in their first year of life by the early 1860s, whereas in Norfolk only the Wayland poor law union attained even a 50 per cent level and some 20 per cent of Norfolk schoolchildren went unvaccinated. These low levels were attributed to the scattered population, to 'the ignorant obstinacy of the poor' and, particularly, to the lack of interest by the local Guardians.[56] Indeed, Dr Buchanan, compiler of the investigation added, 'I have to remark that in some unions they have taken no interest whatever in the subject, beyond occasionally remonstrating at the size of a contractor's account.'[57]

As for the isolation facilities, in 1908 MoH Dr Lack stated publicly that the Forehoe RDC isolation hospital was so inadequate that he might no longer use it and even discharge its existing patients. In response, his local sanitary committee stated that it would consider making improvements, but only commensurate with those facilities that, in 'a small Union can fairly be expected.' It criticised his 'wholly condemnatory' tone, adding that 'it would be folly to expend any sum upon this place if it is to be practically boycotted by its medical officer.'[58] Even when faced with continuing local outbreaks of scarlet fever and diphtheria,

53 Neither of Chadwick's prescriptions, of centralised poor law provision for uniformity and for efficiency gains to be derived from public health investment, found much support within rural local government.

54 J. M Dodds, Report 9 December 1896 and Minute 10 December 1896 in SRO, HH 58.7, in Levitt, (ed.) *Social Conditions in Scotland*, 144.

55 Digby, *Pauper Palaces*, 169.

56 'Dr Buchanan's Summary of the results of his inquiry in Norfolk and parts of Suffolk' in Appendix II, Reports...on the State of Public Vaccination', *Fourth Report of the Medical Officer of the Privy Council 1861*, London, HMSO 1862, 110-130, 110-113.

57 *Fourth Report of the Medical Officer of the Privy Council 1861*, Dr Buchanan, 113.

58 NRO, DC 5/1/1, Forehoe RDC Sanitary Committee, 27 July 1908.

Forehoe RDC remained reluctant to make major improvements or to use its full powers, for example reporting instances in which 'the parents had declined to allow the (child) case to be taken to the isolation hospital, but every precaution had been taken to prevent the spread of disease.' [59]

Yet open conflicts between rural MosH and governing bodies were infrequent, not least because the former also had to consider their social and official positions in relation to the business of making a medical living. Whereas their urban counterparts were usually full-time, with salaries that allowed a degree of independent thinking, rural doctors could not contemplate a career in public health medicine. Their income came primarily from private family doctoring, so they were often compromised in their public health work in relation to local government figures and property owners. As *The Lancet* described in 1872, 'they and their friends were his patients, or potential patients ... A competitive doctor could not afford to alienate respectable members of the parish.'[60] Taking the example of Freebridge Lynn, west Norfolk, Anne Digby noted that 'infectious disease was allowed to spread unchecked, while nuisances flourished without interference. The local guardians had given their medical officer the impression that he was never to act on his own initiative and was to wait for local requests for his intervention, which rarely came.' [61]

When Dr Back, MoH for St Faith's and Aylsham, did report unfit properties and overcrowded cottages, his local sanitary committee was simply informed that the main landlord, 'Lord Orford was not aware of any deficiency of inhabitable cottages and that his own farms were amply supplied.' Subsequently land agent Douglas Smith, representing the principal landowners in the district, simply told the Committee 'that *he* did not consider there was any deficiency of cottage accommodation.' [62] The possibility that enthusiastic doctors might lose

---

59 NRO, DC 5/1/1, Forehoe RDC Sanitary Committee, 22 October 1910.

60 *The Lancet* 1872, cited in Brand, J.L. *Doctors and the State: the British medical profession and government action in public health*, Baltimore, Johns Hopkins Press, 1965, 17. This also reflected professional weaknesses (the Poor Law Medical Officers Association was founded in 1868, but needed support from the British Medical Association in its campaigns) although doctors and the guardians might share similar values. See Crowther, 'Paupers or patients?', 53.

61 Digby, *Pauper Palaces*, 175. Crowther, M.A. *The Workhouse System 1834-1929*, London, Batsford, 1981, 172, made a similar point with reference to poor law doctors and the Guardians. Social deference was often expected: although the Holkham estate had good *mid-19th* c. reputation, the local MoH was still not carrying out inspections in 1919 'because it was well known that cottages in those parishes were in a superior condition, and Lord Leicester had intimated his intention of building whatever further cottages were necessary'. NRO, C/MH1/12b, *Norfolk MoH Annual Report 1919-20*, 31.

62 NRO, DC3/1/23, St Faith's and Aylsham Sanitary Committee Minute Book 1911-22, 46, 52, 142,144. This occurred during 1911-12: there was no resolution before 1914 and the Local Government Board itself was unwilling to offer loans during the World War One.

their office in any confrontation over public health had been anticipated in Scotland from the introduction of the 1867 Act: 'If medical officers are removable at the caprice of the local authorities without culpe (blame) of any kind alleged against them, it would be impossible for them in many cases to do their duty fearlessly and independently... in most of our parochial boards the classes with whom sanitary measures are unpalatable form the majority.'[63]

Some well-meaning sanitary effort was counter-productive, since the condemnation and closure of cottages without replacement frequently meant the eviction of tenants to the workhouse. Thus, after Mr Wilson refused to repair his Wood Dalling cottage in 1911, 'The sanitary committee duly made an Order under section 17 of the Housing Act, 1909 closing the cottage. Notice to give up possession was given to Enoch Wymer on the 22nd September (and) In November Wymer, his wife and children were admitted to the workhouse, having nowhere else to go.'[64] Dr Back similarly reported to Blofield RDC (1908) on a cottage in which

> 'the roof is not altogether weather-proof; the walls and floor are damp ... there is an insecurity about bulging walls; and the bedroom (is) situated in the pitch of the roof with insufficient airspace ... Such a cottage is not worth putting into a proper state of repair (but) to pull it down would only result in depriving a labourer and his family of their only available shelter. I respectfully submit this difficult problem to the consideration of the council'.[65]

In cases such as this, doctors could do little when the political will or resources to provide good affordable rural housing were missing, for although 'rural parish councils frequently asked their district councils to provide housing and just as frequently had their requests turned down ... none seems to have taken up their case with the County Council.'[66] It is of some significance that, even when they had powers to build houses under the 1890 Housing of the Working Classes Act, assisted by loans from the Local Government Board, only Thetford among the

---

63 W.S. Walker, Secretary to the BoS, wrote to the Lord Advocate 16 June 1867 concerning the ease of removal of local medical officers. SRO, AD56/276/2. In Levitt, (ed.) *Social Conditions in Scotland*, 8.

64 NRO, DC3/1/23, St Faith's and Aylsham Sanitary Committee Minute Book, 1911-1922, 29 August 1911, 26. This was a common problem: in 1888 the North Pickenham (Swaffham) MoH singled out seven dilapidated cottages but did not apply the law, knowing that RDC could not afford to build. NRO, C/MH1/7b, 103, 108.

65 NRO, C/MH1/3, *Norfolk MoH Annual Report 1907*, Rural Districts, 3. Similarly Stalham's sanitary inspector noted a 'completely unfit' cottage but, as two rooms were occupied by an elderly invalid, 'I thought it advisable not to ask the MoH to condemn the cottage at present'. NRO, DC 22/3/30 Stalham RDC Inspector's Report, 1912.

66 Linsley, 'Homes for Heroes', 27.

Norfolk local authorities had begun to act before 1914.[67] The equivalent measure in Scotland also had only a limited initial effect from 1890 because the legislative powers to order housing improvements or demolition on public health grounds or to undertake new building had to be specifically adopted by each burgh or local authority and there was considerable reluctance to do this.[68] And while the preparatory 1885 Royal Commission on the Housing of the Working Classes had acknowledged sanitary defects, it was otherwise complacent on the question of housing shortages or the need for general building programmes, even though doctors linked poor and overcrowded housing with rickets, childhood infections, respiratory and intestinal diseases.[69]

A comparison of evidence to the 1832-4 and 1905-09 Poor Law Commissions indicates a growing medical contribution in official discourse, partly reflecting the doctors' sanitary and public health role. Yet this still might be ambivalent or moralistic, particularly if doctors shared the cultural values of the better off. [70] For example, Anne Crowther has suggested that poor law medical officers, 'when their professional duty was clear – as in the treatment of infirmary patients … usually tried to uphold the standards of their profession. When their responsibilities were ambiguous, Poor Law standards might dominate.'[71]

Might the same apply in the doctor's public health role or was there a distinct move towards scientific approaches and medical claims to expertise-based authority? The persistence of sanitarian views regarding campaigns against 'dirt', which often included moral aspects and individual predisposition as qualities to be considered regarding infection, should be acknowledged.[72] Processes of putrefaction and germination might be differently interpreted by sanitarians and bacteriologists and some of those reluctant to adopt a bacteriological approach argued that, just as zymotic diseases were brought under control by improved sanitation, so 'germs' might be. With a clean, healthy environment considered

67 Gauldie, E. *Cruel Habitations: a history of working class housing 1780-1918*, London, Allen and Unwin, 1973, Appendix 4, 322-3. By then 181 local authorities, mainly urban districts, had aquired land or begun to provide public housing.

68 The 1909 Housing, Town Planning etc Act finally applied the 1890 measures on a general basis.

69 Rodger, 'Crisis and confrontation', 25-53, 30.

70 Crowther, 'Patients or Paupers?', 50, suggests that would-be reformers of the English Poor Laws, such as Sidney and Beatrice Webb 'wished to give doctors power to enforce not only public health but public morals ... (these) …views were a logical development from the existing role of the Poor Law medical officer as a disciplinarian'.

71 Crowther, 'Patients or Paupers?', 53.

72 Stevenson, L.G. 'Science down the Drain', *Bulletin History of Medicine* Vol. 29, (1955), 1, 1-26. He cites Owesi Temkin's 1953 depiction of the combination of environmental improvement and a hygienic, goodly life as a nineteenth century 'second secularisation of the concept of infection',.4.

good for individuals and 'bad' for germs, continuing emphasis was placed upon the properties of pure water, sunlight and oxygen levels. [73] Other MosH were pragmatists, believing their own efforts to be 'very far in advance of theory'; Michael Worboys' study suggesting 'they maintained that, despite knowing little or nothing about the intimate nature of 'disease-poisons', they knew how to reduce their spread, violence and effects.'[74] Moreover those doctors with a wider social outlook were also fearful that 'the long struggle to reduce poverty and improve education might be abandoned in the headlong rush to the laboratory' and that the latter would be urban-based, perhaps even depriving the countryside of medical and sanitary practitioners.[75]

In 1869 the first national professional grouping of MosH was established and increasing attention was paid to hygiene and public health issues in medical training from the mid-1880s. [76] In the following decade matters such as disease notification and control; the focusing upon population groups 'at risk' and the importance of laboratory facilities featured more prominently in the work of MosH, who were also likely to emphasise their own expertise and technologies

73 Thus Sir William Job Collins, one time President of the Sanitary Association referred to 'the efficacy of isolation and the limitation of infection, the utility of oxidising disinfectants, the salubrity of the country and morbidity of the town, the success of the cool or open-air treatment of certain diseases, the decline of zymotic diseases before the progress of sanitation.... making our hygiene so good that prophylactics and antiseptics shall be superfluous', *Lancet* 2, 4 December 1880, cited in Stevenson, 'Science down the Drain', 19. Writers in the *Contemporary Review* similarly prescribed the countryside for a wholesome upbringing, bodily physique, rational recreation and convalescence, see Palmengiano, E.M *Health and British Magazines in the Nineteenth Century*, Lanham, Scarecrow Press, 1998; Merivale, C. 'Remarks on the physique of the rural population', *Contemporary Review*, 10, (1869), 265-72; Roberts, C. 'Physiology of recreation', *Contemporary Review* 68 (1895), 103-13.

74 Worboys, M. Spreading *Germs: disease theories and medical practice in Britain 1865-1900*, Cambridge, Cambridge University Press, 2002, 38. Such 'social' medicine might also offset the impact of industrialisation; or enhance the Body Politic or state modernisation projects. See Fee and Porter, 'Public health', 250-1; Raeff, M. *The well-ordered police state... the Germanies and Russia*, New Haven, Yale University Press, 1983, 192, 199.

75 see Hutchinson, J.F. 'Tsarist Russia and the bacteriological revolution', *Journal History of Medicine*, 40, (1985), 420-39, 430. Note that he is referring to *English* sanitarians here.

76 This was the Association of Medical Officers of Health: there were 828 rural and urban MosH in 1876 and 1,770 by 1900 and about one-half were members. The first English Diploma in Public Health (DPH) was offered at Cambridge University in 1875 and the DPH was recognized as a postgraduate medical qualification in 1888, by which time nearly 400 doctors were so qualified. Wohl, A. *Endangered Lives. Public Health in Victorian Britain*, London, J.M. Dent, 1983, 182-4.

in general health promotion, expecting due acknowledgement from the public.[77] The later Norfolk MosH reports, for example, were less suggestive of shared views with landowners or farmers on questions of immorality, drunkenness or filth among rural poor and contained greater criticism of those responsible for health nuisances.[78] But whether as 'nuisance spotters', germ-hunters or (later) as eugenicists, doctors might have other agendas and 'in programmes for inspection of school children, home visitation, education of new mothers, there remained ambiguity over whether the help given by public health workers was in support or accusation'.[79] Consequently such work was sometimes ineffective or risked counter-productive responses, whereas improvements might also reflect features such as familiarity, 'public manners' or sheer optimism. Thus by 1889 in Thetford district, 'the inspector says the people see the advantages of keeping their places in a better condition than in years gone by and that he has no difficulty now in having his orders attended to.'[80] Similarly Norfolk RDC meetings during the 1890s more typically contained comments to the effect that 'the action taken by owners and occupiers respectively for the abatement of nuisances reported be deemed satisfactory.'[81]

Nevertheless, there were also suggestions of more scientific analyses by the early 1900s. For example Dr J.T.C. Nash, Norfolk MoH from 1907, claimed in his first annual report successes for free and preventive antitoxin measures against diphtheria and outlined an anti-typhoid campaign that focused upon water, milk, shellfish and the attempted identification of 'carriers', rather than older-style investigations of defective drains and 'sewer air'. Declining infant mortality rates were linked with hygiene promotion work, involving doctors, public lectures and 'other agencies in the education of working class mothers in

---

77 See Lawrence, C. *Medicine in the making of Modern Britain 1700-1920*, London, Routledge, 1994, 72-3 and Fee and Porter, 'Public health', 269-70. Specialist qualifications were also introduced: an additional requirement in Dr Littlejohn's appointment as part of the Executive assisting the Scottish Secretary was a Diploma in Public Health Medicine. Levitt, *Poverty and Welfare in Scotland*, 24.

78 Burchardt, J. *Paradise Lost: Rural Idyll and Social Change in England since 1800*, 2002, 46-8 notes that middle class aspirations to rural, 'natural' or 'wholesome' surroundings sometimes reflected anxieties over urban environmental and character defects, which some doctors may have shared.

79 Hamlin, C. 'State medicine in Great Britain', in Porter, D. (ed) *The History of Public Health and the Modern State*, Amsterdam, Rodopi, 1994, 132-64, 153.

80 NRO, C/MH1/1 *Norfolk MoH Annual Report 1889*, 43, 108. For Docking RDC that year 30 sanitary notices were issued, along with 45 'mild' inspector's notices; 62 'letter-only' communications and 120 cases 'dealt with by word of mouth', suggesting many minor instances and improvements? Ibid. 43.

81 NRO, Henstead RDC Minutes 1895 - 16 March 1897.

the proper care of infants.'[82] He was similarly attempting to evaluate isolation hospital provision, in response to the perplexing pattern of 'scattered yet clustered' infectious disease outbreaks in rural districts. And a further campaign to avoid the contamination of water courses focused upon the shallow burial of excreta, 'because we depend upon the bacteria in the surface soil to oxidise the excretal products and render them useful for plant life.'[83]

District-level MosH reports also featured greater emphasis upon new technologies, such as 'a steam disinfector in which bedding, clothing, carpets and suchlike can be efficiently disinfected', or the utilisation of superheated steam and spraying of disinfectant solution, rather than older methods of fumigation which was 'far from satisfactory or efficient.'[84] Similarly there was more widespread condemnation of past practices and calls for sweeping reform, notably an end to 'the old fashioned abomination known as the cess pit', and to customs whereby 'our forefathers deemed it necessary to sink their drinking water well within a few feet of their cesspit'. Regrets were also expressed that, alongside the usual instances of new wells, cleared privies or reconstructed drains, there was, as yet, 'nothing *systematic*' (my emphasis SC).[85]

This new awareness reflected professional standards and the influence of technological approaches, prompted by the Royal Sanitary Institute from 1877.[86]

Of course, doctors still revealed ideological differences in their proposed remedies. Thus Norfolk doctor G. P. Cross (MoH Downham) felt that 'there are many houses that ought to be condemned but it will be impossible to do this until they can be replaced', and meanwhile proposed a 'two into one' cottage conversion policy to address overcrowding, pending a publicly-subsidised general housebuilding programme. In contrast, W Royden (MoH Flegg) deplored the numbers of 'two bedroom hovels' but remained convinced that 'private enterprise is gradually effecting a marked improvement in the dwellings of the poor.'[87] In Scotland some doctors, notably Littlejohn and Russell, the MosH for Edinburgh and Glasgow respectively, went further by making direct public appeals in which they 'projected housing and sanitary matters into local newspaper

82 NRO, C/MH1/3 *Norfolk MoH Annual Report 1907* (J.T.C. Nash) 1907, 20. Pamphlets issued to each new mother promoted domestic hygiene, but may also have reflected wider concerns over 'defective mothering', illustrating the ambiguities referred to previously.

83 NRO C/MH1/3 NCC Norfolk MoH, 1907, 24, 34-35.

84 NRO C/MH1/3 NCC Norfolk MoH, 1907. MoH Freebridge, 6; MoH Thetford RDC, 23.

85 NRO, C/MH1/3 *Norfolk MoH Annual Report 1907*, MosH reports: Docking, 6; Depwade, 4; Forehoe, 11.

86 The RSA began as the Sanitary Institute of London in 1876, promoting sanitary engineering, bringing together doctors, engineers and surveyors, and acting as the certifying body for sanitary inspectors. Wohl 1983, p. 194.

87 NRO, C/MH1/3 *Norfolk MoH Annual Report 1907*, MosH reports: Downham, 8, Flegg, 10.

headlines through their reports, lectures and publications ... Raising public consciousness was the first step towards engaging the political will in relation to improved housing standards.'[88]

In still broader contexts it might be argued that the emergence of trades unions, notably the Scottish Miners Federation in Fife, and radical Liberal or Socialist influences were necessary in building up political forces capable of challenging the local dominance of landlordism. This happened in parts of Scotland during World War One, forcing the adoption of wartime rent controls in 1915, the 1917 Royal Commission on Housing and publicly-subsidised housebuilding from 1919, although any Norfolk contribution in this respect was much less discernible.[89] Public health and sanitation issues featured, but not predominantly, in such campaigning, which was itself relatively new.

Given the scope of this paper, its conclusions are less controversial and more modest. Growing medical and other concern with rural health over the second half of the nineteenth century was increasingly expressed in terms of defects in housing, sanitation and the environment, along with the need for more medical personnel with appropriate expertise. Earlier perceptions of the 'healthy rural' marred by the defective habits of countrymen and women changed with modified concepts of personal defect, but were not abandoned. In this respect, proposals for remedial hygiene education, more doctors and their greater influence over emerging services might be ambivalent, rather than representing new objective or scientific approaches, even though they did suggest forms of rural medicalisation in its narrower, profession-orientated sense.[90]

In any event, a medical 'supply-side analysis' focusing upon the doctor's role needs to acknowledge certain realities seen in essentially rural or industrialising areas away from the main urban centres. An interactive perspective acknowledges the efforts of determined medical reformers and their application of scientific advances, but also the obstacles they faced and the likelihood of conflicts of interest. Many rural doctors acting in a public health role had to compromise, considering their own remuneration and the local medical

88 Rodger, 'Crisis and confrontation', 26.

89 Rodger, 'Crisis and Confrontation', 47. The combination of labour militancy and rent strikes in Glasgow in 1915 were particularly important in this respect. In Norwich socialists had some successes in opposing landlords from the early 1900s but the trade union base was weaker here and still more so in agricultural Norfolk. Cherry, S. *Doing Different? Politics and the Labour Movement in Norwich 1880-1914*, Norwich, Centre of East Anglia Studies, 1990, 102-3.

90 While scientific medicine might be equated with novel or urban values, rural doctors often came from established local families. They were thus not necessarily outsiders but might be part of a 'local culture' that was actually marked by social class and lifestyle differences.

marketplace. Moreover, any central state influence or legislation relating to rural sanitation, housing and health was likely to be mediated by those who constituted poor law and local council or burgh authorities, since these had their own interests and were usually more concerned with matters of economy than with the value or benefits of public health reform.

In such contexts, the roles of the doctor as scientific expert or of the sanitary inspector as the designated 'nuisance knower' were limited and variable. Part-time MosH in rural areas were neither in a strong position nor necessarily focused sufficiently upon their public health role, when compared with the full-time urban MosH with greater resources and influence. Just as public access to rural medical practitioners did not depend simply upon *their* availability, but hinged upon questions of social class, affordability, gender and cultural difference, so the doctor's scope as public health official was not merely a matter of expertise and influence, but was largely shaped by local political realities and the requirements of the medical living.

REFORMS AND RURAL HEALTH POLICIES IN REPUBLICAN SPAIN

Josep L. Barona

From the late nineteenth century sanitary reformism became a strong movement in Western countries as a manifestation of progress and modernity, assuming varying forms and levels of action. Strongly rooted in the values and thinking style of the urban bourgeoisie,[1] the hygienic ideology involved programmes of social reformation not only covering health, housing, town planning, diet, schools and public spaces but also aiming to change values and regulate behaviours, characterised by Norbert Elias as the *process of civilisation*.[2] Following a similar perspective Alfons Labisch characterised this as the construction of *homo hygienicus*.[3] Hygienism contributed to a new body culture, reshaping daily life and healthy habits, and to revised concepts of disease and contagion, giving a new meaning to filth and cleanliness, not only in a real sense but also at a symbolic level. As a principal tool of the civilising process, it defined norms and prohibitions that soon became internalised by the population, leading to legal and moral regulations, new values and actions for social reform. The present chapter aims to discuss the origins and historical context of Spanish liberal reforms and the configuration of a sanitary movement to cope with poverty, disease and bad living conditions in urban and rural areas during the last years of the nineteenth century. Special attention is paid to health care reforms in rural districts during the Republican period (1931-1939), in which rural health became a major part of the 'civilising programme' of Spanish society. Reformist policies in rural areas, mainly implemented by liberals and socialists during the biennium 1931-1933, formed an essential part of the modernisation and social regeneration project.

Liberal reforms and the origins of the sanitary movement in Spain

The health status of Western societies in the mid nineteenth century was strongly influenced by the high incidence of infectious diseases. In the case of Spain,

---

1 The concept of *style of thinking* was proposed by the German immunologist Ludwik Fleck during the Inter-war period, applied to a sociological approach to scientific knowledge in his *Einführung in der Genese und Entwicklung einer wissenschaftlichen Tatsache* (1935) a work that clearly inspired Thomas Khun's model on scientific change.

2 Elias, N. *The Civilizing Process, Vol.II. State Formation and Civilization*, Oxford, Blackwell, 1982.

3 Labisch, A. *Homo Hygienicus. Gesundheit und Medizin in der Neuzeit*, Frankfurt, Campus, 1992.

the first decades of the twentieth century correspond to the so-called sanitary and demographic transition. As of the second half of the nineteenth century, health authorities started a process of intervention, including legal and social actions to improve people's health and the targeting of specific groups. Active complicity between hygienists and politicians served to instruct society, spreading hygienic concepts and practices to improve living conditions, particularly in rural areas and workers' districts.

The phenomenon had its international dimensions as it has been pointed out in the introductory chapter of this book. From the *Comité de Salubrité* established in France in 1790 to the *British Sanitary Movement* and the wide dimensions of the German *medizinische Polizei*, an international reformism associated with liberal societies included health as a main factor.[4] In Spain, the hygienist movement was boosted by the reformist liberals from the outset. Mateo Seoane, a liberal exiled in Britain, produced his *Consideraciones generales de estadística médica* (1837) clearly inspired by the ideas of the British sanitary movement. However, the failure of most liberal reforms in nineteenth century Spain delayed the publication of a *Boletín de Estadística Demográfico-Sanitaria de la Península e Islas Adyacentes* until 1879. Subsequent health policies, associated with the civilising process, and the first public health care models reflected the establishment of the bourgeois state and its way of facing periods of crisis and negotiation with the labour movement. In most early twentieth century Western countries the traditional conception of a liberal state based upon *laissez faire* principles experienced a shift, as the state assumed a major role in social and sanitary matters. In this sense a providential state, promoting public politics, social assistance and health care, emerged. As the social and economic advantages of public health interventions became evident, the political dimension of health was accepted.[5] Indeed the emerging providential state during the first half of the twentieth century was in most countries transformed into a welfare state after World War Two.[6]

4 Rosen, G. *A History of Public health*, New York, MD Publications, 1958. An expanded edition: Baltimore, Johns Hopkins University Press, 1993, with an Introduction by Elizabeth Fee and a biographical essay and new bibliography by Edward T. Morman.

5 Salort Vives, S. *Vivir y morir en Alicante. Higienistas e inversiones públicas en salud (1859-1923)*, Alicante, Publicaciones Universidad de Alicante, 2008.

6 Andresen, A. and Grønlie, T. (eds.) *Transferring Public Health, Medical Knowledge and Science in the 19th and 20th Century*, Bergen, Stein Rokkan Centre for Social Studies, 2007; Andresen, A. *et al.* (eds.) *Citizens, Courtrooms, Crossings*, Bergen, Stein Rokkan Centre for Social Studies, 2008; Baldwin, P. *The Politics of social solidarity. Class bases of the European Welfare State 1875-1975*, Cambridge, Cambridge University Press, 1990; Barona, J.L.; Bernabeu, J. *La salud y el estado. El movimiento sanitario internacional y la administración española*, Valencia, PUV, 2008; Swaan, A. De *In Care of the State*, Oxford Polity Press, 1988.

Coping with infectious diseases: the birth of National Institutions

The decrease in general mortality was not uniform during the so-called sanitary and demographic transition. It showed deep differences and different tendencies in rural and urban areas, bourgeois districts and workers' suburbs. Traditionally, urban mortality was higher than in rural districts, with the so-called urban penalty a consequence of migrations and the concentration of unhealthy spaces, houses, hospitals and prisons, in which poverty, disease and exclusion formed into a dreadful triangulation. Environmental contamination and human agglomeration worsened the situation in industrial areas, especially during the second half of the nineteenth century.

The Spanish transition lagged behind that of many other European countries. Infant and child mortality rates were around 245 per 1,000 in the 1860s and 1870s and life expectancy at birth was under 30 years.[7] Child epidemics such as smallpox, measles and diphtheria rose at the end of the nineteenth century, as did intestinal diseases. Epidemiological historians explain this phenomenon as a consequence, to a certain extent, of impaired environmental conditions both in private and public spaces. On the other hand, the incorporation of young women into the industrial workforce changed their traditional role at home – associated with maternity – and disrupted traditional breastfeeding patterns, leading to wet-nursing and artificial feeding. Hygienists immediately saw malnutrition and an unbalanced diet as the source of most health problems among children.

In the closing decades of the nineteenth century, municipal health services were developed in Spain and health officers and chemical and bacteriological laboratories represented the starting point of local health policies and institutions.[8] A state dimension could be seen in the creation of a Directorate General for Health (1899) and national institutions such as the *Instituto Nacional de Sueroterapia, Bacteriología e Higiene Alfonso XIII* (1899) (National Institute of Serotherapy, Bacteriology and Hygiene Alfonso XIII) ; and legislation for the prevention of workplace accidents (1901); the regulation of child labour and women's work (1901); the compulsory vaccination against smallpox, for child protection and the repression of begging (1904), and the General Instruction of Health (1904), among others. Similarly *Institutos Municipales de Higiene* (Municipal Health Institutes) were established in populations exceeding 15,000 inhabitants; milk depots expanded in capital cities, and provincial health brigades and *Institutos Provinciales de Higiene* (Provincial Health Institutes) were established following the 1925 *Reglamento de Sanidad Provincial* (Provincial Health Reglement).

---

7 Salort, 'Vivir y morir', 46

8 Barona and Bernabeu, 'La salud y el estado'.

The expansion of health institutions – mainly in urban areas – preventive campaigns and the improvement of living conditions was stimulated by cultural factors such as the association of hygiene and positive health statistics with modernity. High mortality rates and infant mortality signified intolerable backwardness, an obstacle to wealth and the economy, forcing the upper classes and the state to recognise and to assume the costs of disease. Early twentieth-century Spanish society generally accepted the meaning of the expression '*public health is wealth',* this becoming the starting point for the establishment of a health administration defined in collaboration with the Rockefeller Foundation and influenced by Spanish engagement with international agencies such as the *Office Internationale d'Hygiène Publique,* the League of Nations Health Committee, and International Sanitary Conferences.[9]

Yet the state budget for public health was limited, and sanitary campaigns and health institutions were mostly dependent upon charity. Echoing Max von Pettenkoffer's demonstration of the benefits of public investment in health in Ba-varia, Antonio Espina y Capo, a liberal progressive doctor, presented a paper at the Conference for Social Insurance promoted by the *Ministerio de Fomento* (1917) (Ministry of Development), in which he estimated the cost of excessive avoidable mortality to be five million pesetas for the first decade of the century. Nevertheless, attempts to involve the state in financing health campaigns and institutions often ended in absolute failure, as with Francisco Moliner's political campaigns to promote state construction of a network of tuberculosis hospitals. In 1920 government spending on health amounted to only 0.2 per cent of the national budget, a level trebled only during the *Bienio Reformista* (1931-1933) of the Second Republic.[10]

From the 1880s, liberal reformers supported by a part of the workers' movement set up a *Comisión de Reformas Sociales* (Commission for Social Reforms), which represented a change of mentality in coping with poverty.[11] The promoters, Gumersindo de Azcárate and Segismundo Moret, belonged to the liberal progressivist elite within the bourgeoisie. Against the background of economic and social crisis, new sociological methods and a European reforming impulse – whether Bismarckian programmes or British Fabianism – this proposed initiative represented something completely novel in Spain. In 1883 the liberal government published a project for social reforms looking to reconcile working-

9 Barona and Bernabeu, 'La salud y el estado'.

10 Barona, J.L. *José Chabás Bordehore. Tuberculosis y Medicina Social en la Valencia del primer tercio del siglo XX*, Valencia, Consell Valencia de Cultura, 2008.

11 *Comisión para el estudio de las cuestiones que interesan a la mejora o bienestar de las clases obreras tanto agrícolas como industriales y que afectan a las relaciones entre el capital y el trabajo* [Comisión for the study of matters regarding the improvement or wellbeing of workers classes both peasants and industrial affecting the relations between capital and work].

class and bourgeois interests and it established a commission to identify all matters affecting the improvement and well-being of the working class, peasants and industrial workers included. The *Comisión de Reformas Sociales* was a consultative and technical board, endowed with a central structure and provincial delegations. Its first action was the preparation of a survey based on professional opinions (doctors, teachers, judges, workers, and lawyers) and institutions such as *Institución Libre de Enseñanza, Ateneo Casino Obrero* in Valencia, Faculty of Law and Ateneo in Madrid, among others. However, parts of the labour movement were critical of the initiative: socialist unions criticised the reformist ideology of the commission and the anarchist union did not participate.

Poverty was no longer considered by all liberals as a natural or unavoidable phenomenon threatening social stability. Reformists tried to analyse its causes and dimensions and to involve the providential state in preventive actions and social policies, helping the lower classes and excluded population groups at a time when the rise of urban and industrial concentrations and deteriorating environmental conditions in rural districts were exerting negative consequences on their lives and health.

In public discourse concerning *la cuestión obrera* (the workers' question), political action under the influence of the hygienist movement and the surveys of the *Comisión de Reformas Sociales* was considerable, although the involvement of the liberals in social reformism was also directly linked to fears generated by the increasing strength of the workers' revolutionary movement.

The 1884 *Comisión de Reformas Sociales* survey provided a grim outline, especially regarding malnutrition, poor clothing, housing and the incidence of disease among workers and peasants. Circulation of these findings, the growing influence of the workers' movement, and the boost given by the Berlin Conference to state social interventionism created a positive background for new initiatives.[12] After 1890 the *Comisión* changed its purely consultative status and participated directly in efforts to improve workers' living conditions, a fundamental step in the institutionalisation of social reformism and state intervention in Spain. By 1900 its increased membership included permanent sections devoted to public health and sanitation, focused upon a series of priorities including housing and living conditions, hygiene in factories and schools, and quality control of food and water.

Between 1900 and 1936 the liberal commitment to social matters and the political rise of socialism led to the creation of an *Instituto de Reformas Sociales* (Institute for Social Reforms) in 1903 and the 1908 an *Instituto Nacional de Previsión* (National Institute of Provision), both integrated within the Ministry

---

12 An International Conference was held in Berlin in 1884 to discuss the convenience of State intervention in social matters and the necessity of labour regulations, aspects that were positively supported by the German authorities, Wilhelm II and Bismarck.

of Work and Social Provision in 1920. Similarly, following the Spanish Conference on Social Insurance (1917), social policies included compulsory social security, retirement and labour insurance, and social preventive measures for workers.[13] Many different tendencies – liberal republicans, socialists, regenerationists, anarchists and conservatives – became deeply involved in the extensive programme of social and cultural regeneration.

However, liberal ambiguities concerning state intervention in social reforms and their defence of individual freedom remained, while the social reformists argued that social relations could not be left to private demands. This antagonism over social issues led to a third important group in Spain: the Krausists. These were strong supporters of regeneration and social reform through education and the establishment of an elite committed to progress but, while they supported state intervention, they strongly opposed state intrusion into the autonomous decision-making by individuals, professional associations and institutions from a liberal democratic perspective. Thus only the socialists fully supported the active role of the State as the main social regulator. As we shall see, this opposition to state involvement strongly impinged upon Spanish health policies.

The urban/rural divide: modernisation and backwardness

While rural districts were basically subject to analysis by rural doctors through medical topographies and local health reporting, seeking to attract the attention of health authorities, large towns and cities assumed greater importance and became the focus of health interventions. Unhygienic conditions in workers' houses, chaotic urban planning, and the lack of sanitation and hygienic facilities gave rise to the concept of *social hygiene,* particularly in quality control of water and foodstuffs, cleanliness of streets, public spaces and housing, and health care centres. Architects and engineers were prominent with the *Cuerpo de Ingenieros Civiles* (Body of Civil Engineering), an active and influential liberal reformist group following the establishment of a *Ministerio de Fomento* in 1851 to promote infrastructures and urban projects for the expansion of cities, railways, sanitation and water supplies. At the end of the nineteenth century, the *Revista de Obras Públicas* included a permanent section on Urban Hygiene with a section on Sanitation and Town Planning Expansion later included.[14]

This hygienist civilising movement helped to transform Spain's urban landscape. Urban architects, like Ildeforns Cerdà the architect of the paradigmatic *Eixample* in Barcelona, published a *Demografía estadística de la clase obrera de Barcelona* (1856) (Demographic statistics of the working class in Barcelona) which analysed the deplorable living conditions of workers. With urban improvements underway, attention shifted to the peasants' living conditions, de-

13 Salort, 'Vivir y morir', 93-94.
14 Salort, 'Vivir y morir', 88.

picted as disgraceful by hygienists, architects and rural physicians alike. The advance of medical science would prove useless if the peasantry were not brought into the mainstream of modern civilisation and, as standards of cleanliness were changing, so were political responsibilities for protecting citizens' health. State administration assumed a duty to provide citizens with healthy living conditions. But in Spain and several other European countries the Catholic Church was also a major influence, the line separating religion from politics being imperceptible in modern Spanish history. As Catholic traditionalists saw the emergence of the state in public policies as a transgression of the essence of Spanish tradition, anticlericalism therefore was a key issue for Spanish liberals and republicans. Noticeably, republicans of several ideologies and political orientations were agreed in considering the Catholic Church as the greatest obstacle to progress and modernity in the country.

The Church was especially sensitive and hostile to the intervention of the State and fought against it, still anchored to the charity model and trying to preserve its two traditional roles: instructing the elites and taking care of the poor in a society fundamentally divided into the privileged and the excluded.[15] The Spanish Church did not consider that in the new liberal order the emergent social group might be the middle-class urban bourgeoisie, thus this was not identified as a clearly defined target for its activities. The Church also tried to oppose the role of the State as a social regulator, considering state intervention a threat to its long-standing autonomy and even hegemony in social matters. Consequently, conservative and catholic groups tried to deal with the new social relations through charitable and poor-law mentalities, seeking to counter social reformism, state regulation and intervention.

Rural health becomes a State concern

In September 1930 the Spanish Government officially proposed to the League of Nations Health Committee (LNHC) the convening of a European Conference on Rural Hygiene, an initiative which I have discussed in a previous publication.[16] General concern among hygienists and health administrators over health indicators and living conditions in rural areas had by then been expressed, for example, in the 1923 report published by the Spanish Inspector General for Health

15 Carasa Soto, P. 'Lo privado y lo público en el sistema asistencial: El triángulo Iglesia-Ayuntamiento-Estado en la beneficencia española', in Abreu, L. *Asistencia y Caridad como Estrategias de Intervención Social: Iglesia, Estado y Comunidad (s. XV-XX)*, Bilbao, Servicio Editorial de la Universidad del País Vasco, 2007, 141-172.

16 Barona, J.L. 'The European Conference of Rural health and the Spanish Administration'. In Barona, J.L. and Cherry, S. (eds.) *Health and Medicine in Rural Europe (1850-1945)*, Valencia, PUV, Seminari d'Estudis sobre la Ciencia, 2005, 127-146.

Institutions, Francisco Murillo, on rural health deficiencies.[17] The same concern was reflected in the League of Nations Health Committee joint decision with the Rockefeller Foundation International Health Board in October 1927 to undertake a general survey on health problems in rural Europe. The Spanish authorities as well as other national and international leaders and institutions shared a common preoccupation with the impairment of rural health and living conditions.

During the 1920s hygienists and rural practitioners indicated in a variety of reports and medical topographies the problems regarding health and living conditions in the countryside. The most critical testimonies drew attention to the inadequate application of regulations on slaughterhouses, housing, cemeteries, water supplies and sewage systems, and food control. The municipalities responsible for public health lacked resources; sanitary campaigns were only just underway; the commitment of medical practitioners was mainly to personal or private health care; and the habits of the rural population hindered genuine improvements. Malaria, tuberculosis, venereal diseases, diphtheria, hookworm disease, and trachoma apparently represented unavoidable punishments for Spanish rural populations.[18]

If the Spanish proposal for the European conference was a timely one, it was made more so as significant numbers of industrial workers returned to the countryside as a consequence of the growing economic crisis. Increasing unemployment aggravated poverty and poor living conditions in rural districts. Following preparatory commissions on rural health centres, held in Budapest, October1930, the Conference on Rural Hygiene took place in Geneva in July 1931.[19] It represented a milestone for subsequent reforms in rural health policy in Spain, providing an international context for further initiatives almost concurrently with the proclamation of the Second Republic in April 1931, heralding new reform measures by the incoming socialist government.

Rural health reforms during the biennium 1931-1933

The republican administration regarded health care conditions as deficient and inappropriate for the still largely rural Spanish population. In 1930 almost 60 per cent of Spanish people lived in rural districts, with around 40 per cent in

17 Murillo, F. *De Higiene Rural. Crítica y Alegato*, Madrid, José Góngora Impresor, 1923.

18 Estellés, J. 'Los directores generales de sanidad. Francisco Murillo.' *Boletín Técnico de la Dirección General de Sanidad* (1930), 124-133.

19 Francisco Ruiz Morote published a detailed chronicle: 'La Conferencia de Higiene rural en Budapest', in Pittaluga, G. *La Conferencia Internacional de Higiene Rural convocada por la Sociedad de Naciones (29 Junio 1931)*, Madrid, Publicaciones de la Escuela Nacional de Sanidad (núm. 3), 1931, 43-48.

municipalities containing less than 5,000 inhabitants.[20] In the so-called Reformist Republican Biennium (1931-1933) public health reform was led by socialists who focused on the establishment of a Ministry of Health to coordinate all services by means of a technical centralised organisation. This involved three general directorates: public health, health care, and prevention, and the creation of technical sections dealing with tuberculosis, rural health, children's health, venereal diseases and health statistics, among others. Rural health together with children's health were the principal targets. In effect, the Spanish socialists implemented the conclusions and the models proposed by the League of Nations Conference concerning health care and medical service provision in rural communities and sanitary arrangements in rural districts.[21] These reforms had a preventive agenda and focused on mother-child health protection; the fight against avoidable diseases; the promotion of healthy habits through education and propaganda, and specific sanitary campaigns. The new government also boosted financial support to social medicine, seeking also to develop coordination between medical care and social assistance.

Marcelino Pascua, a specialist instructed at the Johns Hopkins School of Public Health as a fellow of the Rockefeller Foundation, was the Director General for Public Health between April 1931 and May 1933. He was aware of the importance of the rural problem in Spain and focused on an active policy. Professionalisation was a fundamental aim and, under Pascua, new legislation promoted full time dedicated provincial health officers, who were required to give up their private clinical practice.[22] Furthermore, the Provincial Health Institutes (*Institutos Provinciales de Higiene*) – formerly technically dependant on the province – were made answerable to the central Public Health Directorate in Madrid.[23] Drawing upon international experience Pascua also began the reorganisation of national bodies such as the Institute of Health, the Hospital for Infectious Diseases, the School of Health, the School of Maternology and Puericulture, the Institute of Pharmacobiology, the Cancer Institute, and the new School for Visiting Nurses.[24]

---

20 Tuñón de Lara, M. *Tres claves de la Segunda República. La cuestión agraria, los aparatos del Estado, Frente Popular*, Madrid, Alianza editorial, 1985, 22.

21 A detailed analysis of the Geneva Conference on Rural Health, see Barona 'The European Conference', in Barona and Cherry (eds.) *Health and Medicine*, 136-146.

22 *Orden de 17 de junio de 1931 prohibiendo el ejercicio de la profesión médica a los Inspectores Provinciales de Sanidad.*

23 *Decreto de 31 de julio de 1931.* Published at the *Gaceta 2 de agosto de 1931.*

24 Pascua, M. 'La Sanidad pública en el medio rural', El Sol, 14 de abril de 1933, 29; Bernabeu-Mestre, J. *La salut pública que no va poder ser. José Estellés Salarich (1896-1990): una aportació valenciana a la sanitat espanyola contemporània*, València, Consell Valencià de Cultura, 2007.

Centralised coordination of health centres in rural districts was also proposed, utilising the Provincial Institutes of Hygiene (now dependent on the Central Administration) that were considered as tertiary health centres under the European Conference model. These were to lead the technical orientation of the Secondary and Primary health centres operating in each rural district.[25]

Summarising the recommendations of the European Conference and his own experience, the Provincial Health Officer of Valladolid, Francisco Bécares, outlined proposals for the organisation of rural health centres in the province.[26] His scheme was based on the establishment of a *Centro sanitario y de hygiene rural* (Rural Health Centre) in each municipality endowed with a health inspector. This centre would include a *Puesto de socorro de urgencia* (Emergency Aid Post) for simple operations and accident response; a Public surgery for simple medical care; the implementation of preventive campaigns mainly for immunisation against smallpox, typhoid fever and tuberculosis; disinfection activities and a small laboratory for the reception of bodily fluids for analysis and microscopic research. It would also collaborate in campaigns against malaria (detection of insects, analysis of soil, water, and patients) and tuberculosis, through vaccination and propaganda. It would screen the local population to identify TB suspects or those exposed and establish links with more specific anti-tuberculosis dispensaries. Rural health centres were also responsible for the fight against sexually transmitted diseases and the prevention of cancer, leprosy, alcoholism and 'any disease affecting the strength and potentiality of the race'.[27] Maternity and childhood were special subjects of protection through campaigns for the instruction of mothers on child care, breast- and artificial feeding, and school health inspection in collaboration with schoolteachers. Food safety and health administration were also listed among rural centre tasks.

Bécares also acknowledged that improving rural health partly depended upon more general cultural progress, implying a modification of habits.[28] Health administration was to be centralised under a municipal health officer responsible for the co-ordination of health statistics based on empiric records. According to the Bécares project, municipalities were to provide the health centre with the

25 This model was also approved at the First National Conference of Health in Madrid in 1934. Ruesta Marco, S.; Bécares Fernández, F.; Ruiz Morote, F. 'Organización de los servicios de higiene rural. Normas que aconseja la experiencia adquirida para su total desenvolvimiento', in Nágera Angulo, L. (coord.) *Primer Congreso Nacional de Sanidad. Madrid, 6-12 de mayo de 1934*, Madrid, Ministerio de la Gobernación, 1934, col. 1, 235-279.

26 Bécares, F. *Proyecto de nueva organización de servicios sanitarios municipales. Creación de centros sanitarios y de higiene rural*, Valladolid, Publicaciones del Instituto Provincial de Higiene, Talleres tipográficos Cuesta, 1932.

27 Bécares, *Proyecto de nueva organización*, 5.

28 Bécares, *Proyecto de nueva organización*, 3.

necessary infrastructures, which had to be in a clean location, well ventilated and illuminated and endowed with water supply, toilets and a sewage system. Even the internal architecture of the centre was carefully described in his report.

Rural centres were to be divided into three departments, the first catering for the emergency aid post, preventive practices, and laboratory techniques, campaigns against malaria, sexual diseases and administrative activities. A second department dealt with maternity, child care and school inspection, and the third was to offer anti-tuberculosis campaigns and disinfection practices. Larger towns endowed with a service for food control were to have their own premises, including some laboratory facilities. Obviously, the emergency aid post had to have the necessary instruments for simple surgical interventions as well as for vaccination and other preventive campaigns, but health centres were mostly supplied by the Provincial Health Institute, Spain's version of the tertiary health centre. The staff of the primary rural health centre consisted of a medical practitioner with knowledge in social and preventive medicine, a visiting nurse for every six to eight thousand inhabitants, and a health officer devoted to control and vigilance of simple works in sanitation. In the Spanish case, the assistance of *practicantes* – professional health auxiliaries – were considered to be useful.[29] Rural health centres thus became the basic unit of health care and recent research has focused upon their functioning in areas such as Talavera de la Reina and the Valencia province.[30]

In larger towns, Secondary health centres had a similar role but also coordinated their respective primary health centres, organised campaigns against tuberculosis and venereal diseases, trained sanitary staff, and applied simple laboratory techniques. Each had a full-time expert as director, along with visiting nurses, a sanitary engineer, augmented by the services of specialists on the main health problems in the area. Provincial institutes were to supply all the facilities required to take biological products for laboratory analysis, as with water and food samples. Equipment needed by centres in malarial areas would match that in anti-malaria dispensaries, while in anti-tuberculosis dispensaries simple x-ray apparatus was provided. Health instruction and the dissemination of hygienic principles were also central, with pictures, posters, and other propaganda materials targeting the public.

The first decision of the Republican government was to approve a budget for the establishment of 15 secondary centres of rural health in 1932. An Order of 22nd July 1932 announced the appointment of directorates for 15 more rural

29 Pittaluga, *Trabajos de la Conferencia Internacional de Higiene Rural*. Madrid, Publicaciones de la Escuela Nacional de Sanidad, 1931, 41.

30 See: Barona Vilar, C. *Las políticas de la salud*, Valencia, PUV, 2005; Atenza Fernández, J.; Martínez Pérez, J. (eds.) *El centro secundario de higiene rural de Talavera de la Reina y la sanidad española de su tiempo*, Toledo, Junta de Castilla-La Mancha, 2001.

health centres, sanctioned by an Order of 3rd February 1933. Yet these 30 secondary centres fell some way short of Pasqua's estimate of 180 to 200 needed for the rural population within the decade.[31] Municipal cooperation and local financial support were expected to enhance such expansion once local authorities recognised the positive impact of rural health centres on living conditions and the economy of their areas. A second important aspect was the collaboration of rural medical practitioners and municipal health officers in charge of primary health centres with other professionals – practitioners, nurses, surgeons, veterinaries, pharmacists – in rural districts.

The financial cost of the rural health program was estimated by J. Morote, another fellow of the Rockefeller Foundation and a member of the Spanish Commission in the European Conference and Provincial Health Officer in Cáceres.[32] The professionalisation and full-time engagement of the sanitary staff was critical, and good salaries were needed to attract committed staff. Success usually depended upon professional willingness, as municipalities often lacked the funds for health centre infrastructure or ambitious projects and only specialised equipment, such as X-ray apparatus or laboratory materials, was contributed directly by the State. Conceived as the nucleus of positive local transformation in association with improved living conditions, it was hoped that rural health centres would help to dignify peasants' lives and encourage the return of the unemployed from cities and industrial areas due to the growing of unemployment in industrial and urban areas.

A case study: Rural Health Reforms in Valencia Province

From 1928 the monthly *Boletín Sanitario de la Provincia de Valencia* (Health Bulletin of Valencia Province) provided statistics on morbidity and mortality rates from infectious diseases for roughly 150 municipalities in the Province. This compilation was considered essential in developing public health policy. That year the Valencian Provincial Institute of Hygiene offered six prizes to rural practitioners for the promotion of maternal hygiene in pregnancy, delivery and childrearing, respectively *Puericultura* and *Maternología.* An extensive campaign in favour of breastfeeding also aimed at reducing infant mortality during the first year of life.[33] The establishment of a local and provincial

31 Jiménez Lucena, I. 'La Segunda República, una apuesta por la higiene rural: el nivel legislativo', in *Actas del XXXIII Congreso Internacional de Historia de la Medicina. Granada-Sevilla, 1-6 Septiembre 1992*, Sevilla, 1994, 567-580.

32 Morote, J. 'Informe sobre el coste de la Organización Sanitaria de un Distrito Rural', in *Trabajos de la Conferencia Internacional de Higiene Rural*, Madrid, Publicaciones de la Escuela Nacional de Sanidad, 1931, 90-91.

33 *Boletín Sanitario de la Provincia de Valencia*, año II, (1928), num. 10, febrero, 13. The prizes consisted of a financial remuneration of 200 pesetas and the award of a diploma.

administration based on health officers thus encouraged a strategy of civilisation, cent-red on changing domestic habits mainly among housewives. Similarly in April 1928 the Valencian Provincial Board organised a series of lectures on rural health promoted by a national association of municipal health officers, mainly addressed at health professionals but open to the whole population.[34]

The pages of the *Boletín Sanitario* reveal the level of coordination by the Provincial Institute, particularly when acute problems appeared and the rural facilities could not respond quickly. Some actions focused on prevention by means of bacteriological technologies while other measures were mainly centred on the introduction of hygienic patterns in public health. [35] Thus a letter from the Provincial Inspector of Health to the municipalities reflected the instructive and civilising orientation of the rural health programme:

> '... all this has much hygienic importance, because [waste] facilitates the multiplication of flies and mosquitoes, with great damage to public health due to their intervention in the propagation of several diseases: typhoid fever and intestinal diseases, malaria etc., furthermore disturbances produced by putrefaction of organic substances and the ugliness of a dirty town, full of dung all around ... As a consequence of the arguments described we trust that City councils will organize the public cleaning in an efficient way, avoiding dung deposits and sweepings in the proximities of the populations and will demand of whom it may concern the maintenance of irrigation channels and small drains in such a way that they are not a source of mosquitoes.'[36]

During the reformist biennium the coordinating action of the Provincial Health Institute with regard to the rural practitioners and health centres became wider and stronger. The 1928 film *Valencia Protectora de la Infancia* (Valencia protecting children, 1928) was promoted by the School of Puericulture in rural areas in popular campaigns by the *Cátedra Ambulante de Puericultura* (Travelling Chair of Puericulture),[37] and rural districts periodically published reports on their local health and living conditions.[38] The School of Puericulture offered free

34 For example, J. Pérez Feliu lectured on 'La tuberculosis y los tuberculosos en el medio rural', *Boletín Sanitario de la Provincia de Valencia,* año II, (1928), num. 12, abril, 1. [Tuberculosis and tuberculosis patients in rural districts].

35 Martínez Sellés, M. 'Una epidemia de fiebre tifoidea en Loriguilla', *Boletín Sanitario de la Provincia de Valencia,* año II, (1928), núm. 14, 3-4. It tells the positive effects of a massive, preventive vaccination applied to the population of Loriguilla to face an acute outbreak of typhoid fever.

36 *Boletín Sanitario de la Provincia de Valencia,* año II, (1928), núm. 15, agosto, 11-12.

37 *Boletín del Instituto de Higiene de la Provincia de Valencia,* año 5, (1931).

38 Aspectos de la Sanidad rural. Memoria sanitaria de Sollana. Memoria Sanitaria del año 1930.- Distrito de Sueca.- Pueblo de Sollana. Provincia de Valencia.- Habitantes según el

courses to young women, including lessons and visits to child protection institutions while mothers in rural districts were targeted using sanitary booklets containing advice on children's health care.[39] There were also specific campaigns dealing with typhoid fever and trachoma.[40]

Under new regulations from 1931 rural health centres were accountable to the central administration and provincial health officers were forced to develop their job on a full-time basis, private practice being prohibited. Prizes for rural practitioners continued, mostly to recognise their role in the protection of children's health campaigns.[41] Later editions of the *Boletín Sanitario del Instituto de Higiene de la Provincia de Valencia* (Health Bulletin of the Health Institute of Valencia Province) included local reports on health facilities, living and health conditions in several rural areas of the province, some critical but others outlineing the positive results of combining hygienic instruction and adequate health care, which apparently led to refinements in epidemiological records.[42] The *Boletin* also disseminated information on national and international rural health topics, such as the Geneva conference and work done by the National Schools of Hygiene on issues such as milk availability; the fight against infections transmitted by water; rural housing; the treatment of dung and fertilizers; epidemiological records, and financial requirements.

Conclusions

Rural health became a major part of the civilising programme in Spain during the early twentieth century, especially through the reformist policies implemented by liberals and socialists during the first years of the Second Republic. Health, education and the hygienic transformation of the rural formed part of the

---

último censo, 3.621. *Boletín del Instituto de Higiene de la Provincia de Valencia,* año 5, (1931).

39 'La lucha contra la mortalidad infantil. Consejos a las madres que en forma de cartillas sanitarias deben repartirse por los pueblos sobre la crianza y salud de los niños de pecho.' *Boletín del Instituto de Higiene de la Provincia de Valencia,* año 5, agosto, (1931), 9-10.

40 Abril, 1933, 71: 'Consejos prácticos. Profilaxis de la fiebre tifoidea' *Boletín del Instituto de Higiene de la Provincia de Valencia,* año 7, (1933), 1-2; Rubio Huerta, Lorenzo 'El problema social del tracoma. El tracoma y la escuela'. *Boletín del Instituto de Higiene de la Provincia de Valencia,* año 7, (1933), 2-4; Vidal Jordana, Dr. 'La fiebre tifoidea y su mortalidad en la provincia de Valencia.' *Boletín del Instituto de Higiene de la Provincia de Valencia,* año 7, (1933), 68, p. 4-7); Rubio Huerta, Lorenzo 'El problema social del tracoma. La lucha contra el tracoma en la provincia de Valencia.' *Boletín del Instituto de Higiene de la Provincia de Valencia,* año 7, febrero, (1933), 69, 3-4; Fernández Aldave, L. 'El problema social del tracoma. Ideas generales: importancia y gravedad del tracoma.' *Boletín del Instituto de Higiene de la Provincia de Valencia*, año 7, (1933), 70, 5.

41 Boletín del Instituto de Higiene de la Provincia de Valencia, año 5, 49, (1931), 49, 13.

42 Bosch Marín, J. 'Ejemplo digno de imitarse. ¿Se puede hacer *sanidad* en el medio rural?' *Boletín del Instituto de Higiene de la Provincia de Valencia*, año 7, (1933), 78, 1-2.

modernisation and social regeneration project of influential groups of liberal Krausists and socialists. A new category of agents was involved, including health officers, public health experts, bacteriologists, school teachers and doctors, nurses, architects, engineers and politicians. Further, the European Conference on Rural Health gave external legitimacy to Spanish rural health reforms.

Since rural practitioners constantly reported an insufficiently civilised way of life in rural districts, propaganda, hygienic instruction, medical action and sanitary campaigns were mobilised to contribute to changing habits and improving health, seeking to shift the peasantry from backwardness into civilisation. The fight against avoidable diseases included trachoma, malaria, tuberculosis, venereal diseases and alcoholism. Rural health centres became key institutions, with housing, schools, and mother-child relations the main fields of action. Rural districts were also included in the traditional public health policies involving hygienic control of water, food, public spaces such as slaughterhouses, cemeteries, lavatories and markets, and private life: housing, diet and habits. In this sense the State sought to transform peasants into citizens, providing all with the means for a healthy way of life.

However the fight between the State and the Catholic Church provoked deep divisions between liberal, socialists, workers' unions and other freethinkers, and conservatives or traditionalists. From 1934 until December 1935 a new political period – *The Black Biennium* – saw a new Conservative government curtail reformist health policies, transferring health services to the Ministry of Work under the Act for Sanitary Coordination of April 1934.[43] The health budget was substantially reduced and the establishment of rural centres curtailed, with only 14 new additions with reduced staffing. The very continuity of primary health centres was questioned, given the conservatives' preference for private practice medicine. However, the Popular Front, made up of socialists, communists and workers' unions – anarchists included – won the elections in February 1936. Santiago Ruesta, appointed Health Sub-secretary, reactivated the League of Nations model for rural health care, boosting rural centres and providing financial support for staff and facilities.[44] The military coup of July 18th 1936, the ensuing three years of civil war, and its consequences in the Franco dictatorship, Spain's isolation and post war crisis, resulted in a completely different context in which rural health lost its prominence.

43 Jiménez Lucena, 'La Segunda República', 574.

44 For example, 57 posts for heads of centres and health instructors were announced. Orden de 24 de marzo de 1936 (Gaceta de 26 de Marzo); Orden de 30 de Abril de 1936 (Gaceta de 8 de Mayo).

THE RURAL HEALTH BUREAU: AN UNSUCCESSFUL ATTEMPT AT PUBLIC HEALTH SURVEILLANCE IN 1910S SPAIN

Esteban Rodríguez-Ocaña

Recent work by J. Barona, J. Bernabeu, E. Perdiguero and colleagues within this network has established rural health as a main topic within Spanish historiography.[1] My contribution here examines an interesting but little-known initiative, the Rural Health Bureau (*Inspección de Sanidad del Campo,* hereafter RHB), which was active between 1910 and 1918. The Bureau had two original features; first, it was created to focus specifically on rural areas, but as territory outside the authority and responsibility of the *Dirección General de Sanidad* (National Health Department). Second, it prefigured a scheme for total health surveillance in those areas, which was relatively ambitious in scope and included both diseases and environmental and social conditions. It can be seen as highly representative of the Spanish Liberal tradition of seeking information as the main approach to social problems and illustrates the blind alley to which this might lead.

Spanish historiography has summarily depicted the Rural Bureau as a failure, starting with the charge of 'evident inefficiency' in the Royal decree that brought it to an end, which was signed by Francisco Cambó, Minister in a Conservative government of Antonio Maura.[2] Similarly Rico-Avello, a post-war public health officer who compiled a detailed report on the development of Spanish public health administration during the first 25 years of the twentieth

---

1 See Barona, J.L and Cherry, S. (eds.) *Health and Medicine in Rural Europe (1850-1945)*, Valencia, PUV, Seminari d'Estudis sobre la Ciencia, 2005. Also, Granjel, M. *Las Hurdes, el país de la leyenda: entre el discurso ilustrado y el viaje de Alfonso XIII*, Lleida, Editorial Milenio, 2003; Barona, J.L. 'Condicions de vida a l'horta valenciana. El testimoni dels metges', *Afers*, 19 (2004), 67-92; Barona, J.L. '*Health, medicine and cultural interaction in rural Spain 1875-1936*', International Journal of Regional and Local Studies, series 2, 2(2006), 31-51; Bernabeu-Mestre, J. 'Medio urbano y salud en el proceso de modernización. Los trabajos de la Academia de Higiene de Cataluña, 1892-1922', in Beascoechea, J.M.; González, M.; Novo, P.A. (eds.) *La ciudad contemporánea, espacio y sociedad*, Bilbao, Universidad del País Vasco, 2006, 183-200; Galiana, M. E.; Bernabeu-Mestre, J. 'El problema sanitario de España: Saneamiento y medio rural en los primeros decenios del siglo XX'. *Asclepio*, 58/2(2006), 139-164; Rodríguez-Ocaña, E.; Menéndez-Navarro, A. 'La tardía intervención higiénica en el medio rural español: el caso de la lucha contra la anquilostomiasis, 1910-1960', *La Mutua*, 2ª época, n. 16 (2006), 71-86.

2 Royal Decree [herafter, RD] Mº Fomento. *Gaceta de Madrid* [hereafter, *Gaceta*] Oct 26, 1918, 282.

century, described the RHB as a 'disloyal competitor' to the official Public Health structure under the Ministry of Home Affairs, 'an undeserved mockery' and a reason to stifle 'true' public health activities.[3] Earlier critics can also be found among public health experts in the 1920s, including Gustavo Pittaluga and Marcelino Pascua, who worked on anti-malaria campaigns and pointed out methodological shortcomings and factual errors in the statistics produced by the Bureau. Contemporary historians have not advanced beyond these judgements and have depicted it as a wholly negative, bureaucratic undertaking, with no glimpse of any positive aspects.

Whilst initially sharing these views, my research on the history of work diseases unearthed evidence of the impact of the RHB on the development and implementation of the first set of prophylactic measures against hookworm disease in mining. This represented the very first State intervention for the purposes of public health protection in the inner functioning of an industry, yet it appeared to have been expunged from the historical record. [4] A systematic search for the remaining testimonies related to the RHB has included sources in the area of agriculture and development, beginning with the official newspaper (*Gaceta de Madrid*).[5] The national archives (*Archivo General de la Administración)* do not appear to hold any documents related to the Bureau, but there are numerous articles and testimonies of interest in the *Boletín de Agricultura técnica y económica* (Bulletin of technical and economic Agriculture), the official newspaper of the General Directorate for Agriculture, Industry and Commerce from 1909. The library of the old Provincial Hospital in Granada contains a large number of supplementary bulletins published between 1910 and 1918 in the *Revista de Medicina y Cirugía Prácticas* (Journal of Practical Medicine and Surgery), *Revista Iberoamericana de Ciencias Médicas* (Iberian-American Journal of Medical Sciences) and *Gaceta Médica Catalana* (Catalan Medical Gazzette), and *Medicina Ibera* (Iberian Medicine) (from its launch in 1917). Collectors of these bulletins have usually kept only the scientific parts. *El Siglo Médico* (Medical Century), the most widely used source for this period, appears to have been carefully examined by Rico-Avello.[6] This chapter depicts the aims, accomplishments and failures of the Rural Health Bureau as recorded in these sources, beginning with its structure and functions, followed by discussion of its contribution to the state of the rural population's health, and concluding with some thoughts on its political framing and the causes of its demise.

---

3 Rico-Avello, C. *Historia de la sanidad española*, 1900-1925, Madrid, 1969, 55-57 and 177-179.

4 Rodríguez-Ocaña, E.; Menéndez-Navarro, A. 'Higiene contra *la anemia de los mineros*. La lucha contra la anquilostomiasis en España, 1897-1936', *Asclepio, 58*/1 (2006), 219-248.

5 Accessible at http://www.boe.es/aeboe/consultas/bases_datos/gazeta.php

6 Rico-Avello, 'Historia de la sanidad'.

A start for rural public health

In November 1910, the Rural Health Bureau was created within the General Directorate for Agriculture of the *Ministerio de Fomento* (Ministry of Development) in a Liberal government led by José Canalejas.[7] It therefore had a defined relationship with other administrative bodies in this sector, including *Consejos provinciales de Fomento* (Provincial Councils for Development) and *Granjas-Escuela* (Farm-Schools) active in the provinces. However, it had no link with the national public health administration (the three *Inspecciones Generales de Sanidad* and local and provincial health boards) established by the General Health Instruction of 1904 under the *Ministerio de la Gobernación* (Ministry of Home Affairs).[8]

The RHB was originally intended to carry out 'all actions of the state in regard to hygiene and salubrity of the soils, sub-soils and waters in rural districts and areas' in order to prevent endemic and transmissible diseases. These 'actions of the state' were more accurately defined as 'public works' but the objective required the addition of medical expertise to the technical (engineering) expertise already incorporated into agronomical services. It completed the coverage of environmental health matters by the Ministry of Development, which included the fight against locust plagues (begun in 1888, modified in 1908), [9] the Animal Health Bureau (created under the Ministry of Home Affairs in 1899 and transferred to Development in 1907-08), [10] and responsibilities for the health of the travelling public on boats and railroads. [11]

The reasons for creating the new office were set out in the 1910 Royal Decree and in the first general report of its Chief Officer in 1912. Both started by acknowledging the end of the 'healthy rural life', saying for example that 'the healthy qualities of the countryside are illusions', and that 'soils and subsoils are unclean, air and water are impure, food is not always safe and dwellings are not healthy'. [12] Some quantitative evidence was included in the 1910 text, which

7 RD Mº Fomento. *Gaceta*, Nov 26 1910, 459-461.

8 On the forming and development of a national public health administration see Rodríguez-Ocaña, E.; Martínez Navarro, F. *Salud pública en España: de la Edad Media al siglo XXI*, Granada, Escuela Andaluza de Salud Pública (Nueva Salud Pública; 1), 2008.

9 Buj Buj, A. *El Estado y el control de plagas agrícolas. La lucha contra la langosta en la España contemporánea*, Madrid, Ministerio de Agricultura, Pesca y Alimentación, 1996.

10 According to legal provisions as the following: Royal Order (hereafter, RO) Mº de la Gobernación. *Gaceta*, Feb 2 1899, p. 399; R.D. Mº Fomento. *Gaceta*, Oct 31 1907, 392-404; RO (Mº Fomento) *Gaceta*, Feb 16 1908, 668; [Dirección general de Agricultura, Industria y Comercio.- Personal.] *Gaceta*, Dec 31 1908, 1303.

11 RR OO Mº Fomento. *Gaceta*, Jul 14 1911, 187; Aug 30 1911, 567-569; Nov 18 1911, 369; Aug 20 1912, 399; Sep 19 1912, 671 and Oct 4 1912, 39.

12 Sanidad del Campo. *Parte de la Memoria del Director general de Agricultura, Minas y Montes é Informe que el Inspector general de Sanidad del Campo eleva como resultado de*

cited official 1907 statistics ascribing 25 per cent of all deaths and the loss of 24 million working days to 'water- or earth-borne diseases'.[13] Data in the 1912 Report pointed to a 'national impoverishment' that was also demonstrated by the depopulation of certain regions and falls in land prices. The need to restore rural health was considered a national goal because rural areas were still regarded as the main drivers of population growth. Accordingly, making the countryside healthy would increase the strength of the state and, crucially, the economy. The reduction of rural diseases would increase the number of active workers, and extensive drainage would contribute to raising the land prices. Finally, cholera was menacing the Mediterranean shores at that time, providing an immediate reason for action and, indeed, a small cholera outbreak the following year in a few villages of Tarragona province was successfully controlled. The 1912 report cited international models in support of the union between public health and civil engineering work, including the Belgian Rural Health Inspectorate, the US Department of Agriculture Health Service, and Italian anti-malaria legislation.[14]

Thus the main argument in favour of this new body was the economic dimension of rural health problems, the true rationale for the incorporation of health concerns within the general frame of capitalistic governance. This was also the principal underlying force in the rise of social medicine in Europe generally, as in Spain.[15] The creation of the Bureau also exposed the failure of the existing public health organisation under the Ministry of Home Affairs, which from 1904 was responsible for health risk surveillance, hence the open hostility to the new organisation expressed by public health officers and authorities. The RHB was provided with a novel regional structure staffed by 16 officers, who were all physicians who had previously worked in rural practice, had laboratory training in water analysis and had completed one year of studies abroad. The central office was assigned two extra officers as assistants to the chief officer and all were physicians with ongoing clinical practices.

Official regulations for the functioning of the Bureau were formally issued in 1913 and in 1916 under Rafael Gasset as Minister of Development, preserving its features while placing it more firmly within the general Agriculture administration.[16] The regional officers were originally given a place in the regional

---

la inspección que ha practicado en las regiones de Castilla la Vieja, Leonesa, Galicia y Asturias, Extremadura, Andalucia y parte de Levante. Madrid, Ricardo F. de Rojas, 1912, 5.

13 In Spanish, 'enfermedades hídricas y telúricas'.

14 Sanidad del Campo. *Parte de la Memoria...*, 1912, 8-12.

15 Rodríguez Ocaña, E. *La constitución de la Medicina Social como disciplina en España, 1884-1923*, Madrid, Ministerio de Sanidad y Consumo, 1987. Rodríguez-Ocaña, E. 'Medicine as a Social Political Science: The Case of Spain c. 1920', *Hygiea Internationalis*, 7 (2007), 37–52.

16 RR.DD. Mº Fomento. *Gaceta*, Oct 22 1913, 140-147 and Aug 11 1916, 309-317.

farm-schools, with the right to use their laboratory facilities, and it was clarified in the 1916 regulations that they came under the authority of the chief engineers at the farm-schools.

The goals of the new Bureau were legally defined as the study, investigation, proposal to the Ministry of Development and subsequent control of all reforms and necessary works to avoid the causes of the unhealthy state of the rural regions and prevent the spread of water-borne diseases.[17] The Government sought by this means to establish a plan for public works in the countryside that was sustained by a public health rationale. These works could be ordered by the RHB itself, although there seems to be no evidence of this in practice, or by the municipal, provincial or national authorities and were to be supported by a programme run by RHB officers to teach and spread information on health among regional populations, the first time that a health administration had been given this responsibility. Subsequent regulations published in 1913 limited this activity to formal lectures at the farm-schools following a previously approved programme and public talks in villages under inspection.[18]

In June 1911, the Chief Officer announced that the RHB would become a major information-gathering operation, undertaking a general health survey with questionnaires on malaria, drinking water, rural workers' diet, Malta fever and hookworm disease.[19] Further investigations into economic and cultural activities in the countryside and into work-related diseases and rural housing were promised for a near future that never arrived.

Completion of the highly detailed questionnaires was a very laborious task. There was a separate schedule for each issue and for each village or town, including even malaria surveys for every railroad station, and most of the data could only be retrieved after painstaking empirical research. They were administered by the local authorities, although RHB officers had to control and verify the responses and sometimes had to carry out research (e.g., water analysis) themselves. The questionnaire on food and diet, to take an example, was eight pages long and gathered data on the number of peasants and workers in the area and their average salaries and on all types of foods (vegetables, fish and meat, animal products like milk or cheese), including canned food, condiments and drinks, collecting information on prices and on production and consumption per person and per landless peasant. Information was also gathered on dietary habits, the quantity and quality of food intake, types of cooking, eating habits, work practices (in terms of calorie consumption), experience of fraudulent practices, and food and drink-related diseases. Responses were compiled at the Central Office by using an American administrative system of cards, assigning an index

---

17 R. D. Mº Fomento. *Gaceta*, Nov 26 1910, 459-461; art. 3.
18 Art. 47, R.D. Mº Fomento. *Gaceta*, Oct 22 1913, 145.
19 R.O. Mº Fomento. *Gaceta*, Jul 17 1911, 209-231.

number to each town.[20] Personal experience from officials, provincial authorities of all kinds and unidentified physicians were the sources of information, as recorded in some of the published reports.[21]

The activities of the Rural Health Bureau

While national data on malaria and on water resources was compiled, other specific national goals were not accomplished.[22] Partial surveys were completed on hookworm disease in one region,[23] nutritional habits in two regions,[24] and diet-related diseases in the province of Barcelona.[25] The Catalonian regional officer, José Suárez, also wrote a series of articles on work diseases related to rice and hemp cultivation.[26]

---

20 I have been unable to find any remaining examples of these cards besides those already published.

21 See for instance Selma, J. 'Generalidades sobre el Archipiélago Canario, en relación con la Sanidad del campo' *Bol. Agric. Tec. Econ.*, 1911: 929-946 (933).

22 Data on malaria were published for 1912, 1913, 1916 (abridged) and 1918. See: 'Sanidad del Campo. Organización y servicios'. *Bol. Agric. Tec. Econ.* 1917; [July, nº 103], 612-619; Suárez de Figueroa, J. 'El paludismo en Cataluña. Cuadros estadísticos del paludismo en Cataluña durante los años 1912, 1913 y 1915'. *Gac Méd Catal* 1917 (nº 961, Jul 24), 26; 'El paludismo en España. Cuadro estadístico (1913)'. *Gac Méd Catal*; 1917 (nº 964, Sep 8), 142; Inspección de Sanidad del Campo. *Avances de los inventarios de Paludismo y Aguas Potables. Datos remitidos por los Inspectores Regionales*. Madrid, Ministerio de Fomento. Dirección General de Agricultura, Minas y Montes, 1918. On water, reports were published in 1915 [Inspección de Sanidad de Campo. 'Avances del inventario de aguas potables'. *Boletín* suplemento al nº 1385, *Revista de Medicina y Cirugía Prácticas*, Nov 1915, 75-76], in 1916 ['Sanidad del Campo. Organización'], and 1918 [Inspección de Sanidad del Campo. *Avances…*].

23 De la Cuadra, Bonifacio. 'Anquilostomiasis'. *Bol. Agric. Tec. Econ.* 1911, 1049-1052.

24 Selma, J. 'Generalidades sobre el Archipiélago Canario, en relación con la Sanidad del campo'. *Bol. Agric. Tec. Econom.* 1911, 929-946; Colmenares, I. G. 'Apuntes para un estudio de la ración alimenticia normal del obrero del campo'. *Bol. Agric. Tec. Econom.* 1914; [Sep, nº 69], 833-838.

25 Suárez de Figueroa, J. 'Enfermedades determinadas por la alimentación en el obrero agrícola de la provincia de Barcelona durante el año 1916. Morbilidad'. *Gac. Med. Catal.*, 1917; 40/2, 365-367.

26 Suárez de Figueroa, José. 'Las neuritis de los obreros de los arrozales'. *Rev. Med. Cir. Pract.*, CVIII, nº 1372 (1915); 'Descripción clínica de las neuritis de los obreros de los arrozales'. *Rev. Med. Cir. Pract.*, CVIII, nº 1373 (1915), 169-172; 'Algunos datos para el conocimiento de la geografía médica de la "neuritis de los obreros de los arrozales" en Cataluña'. *Rev. Med. Cir. Pract.*, CVIII, nº 1379 (1915), 412-413; 'Los pequeños síntomas de las neuritis de los obreros de los arrozales'. *Rev. Med. Cir. Pract.*, CIX, nº 1382 (1915), 49-50; 'Distintos trabajos en el cultivo del arroz y su relación con las neuritis. Gráficos de las neuritis'. *Rev. Med. Cir. Pract.*, CIX, nº 1390 (1915), 370-372. 'Las neuritis de los arrozales en las mujeres'. *Gac. Med. Catal.*, 39/1 (31 de mayo) (1916), 361-363;

What did this output amount to in practice? The 1912 anti-hookworm law, amended in 1916, represented the first legislation against a work-related disease concerning miners (in practice, only males) and it met the best international standards of the day, even though its practical value was undermined by poor government implementation and its lack of focus on miners' families.[27] Although water and malaria were RHB priority areas, the importance given to nutritional data increased over time. One of the earliest regional reports in 1911 dealt with nutrition in the Canary Islands; another, on the Valencia and Murcia region, was published in 1914. In 1915, the General Officer issued 'preliminary technical information' on the standardization of data gathering on this issue and reported the collection from more than half of the of the municipalities.[28] The Department of Agriculture of the Ministry of Development simultaneously published a complementary leaflet that reproduced the 1914 Valencian survey.[29] A lecture on human diet by the Catalonian physician J. Raventós at the Valencia region farm-school was also published in 1915.[30] At this time the high costs of living caused by World War One led to the first general strike, called jointly by the anarchist (CNT) and the socialist unions (UGT) in December 1916. The passing of a Food Act in November that year failed to contain the unrest[31], which continued despite the organization in 1917 of a *Comisaría General de Abastecimientos* (National Food Bureau), upgraded to Ministry status for the next two years.

The purpose of the surveys was not simply to gain epidemiological knowledge: rather, they aimed to draw attention to the economic dimension of unhealthy rural conditions. In the case of malaria, the data depicted a constant but variable burden of 233,000-301,000 annual cases, their estimated costs rising from 72 to 134 million pesetas, including the price of quinine, unpaid wages and the monetary value of lost lives, calculated on the basis of payments made by conscripts to avoid military duty.[32] These health accounting techniques served to

---

'Alteraciones nerviosas de los obreros trabajadores del cáñamo'. *Rev. Med. Cir. Pract.*; CXIII, nº 1438 (1916), 361-363.

27 Rodríguez-Ocaña, Menéndez-Navarro, 'Higiene contra *la anemia*'.

28 'Alimentación del obrero del campo. Datos técnicos preliminares'. *Bol. Agric. Tec. Econ.*, nº 86, Feb 1915, 141-151.

29 Ministerio de Fomento. Dirección General de Agricultura, Minas y Montes. *Alimentación del obrero del campo: apuntes para su estudio*. Madrid, Imprenta de Ricardo F. de Rojas, 1916.

30 Raventós, J. *Alimentación del hombre*, Valencia, Consejo Provincial de Fomento, 1915. There is a later edition as *Alimentaciò humana*, Barcelona, Mancomunitat de Catalunya, 1923.

31 Ley del Ministerio de Estado. *Gaceta*, Nov 12 1916, 385-387.

32 On the calculation of the monetary value for human life in Spain, see Rodríguez-Ocaña, E. 'El valor económico de la salud', in *La constitución de la Medicina Social*, 20-22.

highlight the costs of health problems and support proposals for reforms, indicating the immediate benefits that they could achieve. It was claimed that the sanitation of areas affected by malaria would increase rural wealth (defined by land prices) by 248 per cent. Thus, water-related diseases, mainly linked to the poor condition or absence of water channels or pipes, were estimated to cost around 33 million pesetas per annum in terms of working days lost and deaths. Based on a price of around 88 million pesetas, investment in water supply improvements might therefore yield an annual interest rate of 38 per cent.[33]

Despite doubts as to the complete accuracy of these very extensive reports, they represented the largest compilation of public health-related environmental data ever produced in Spain: the closest comparison is the production of national death statistics from 1900. The key questions are how they were used and to what ends. It is clear that the laborious gathering of data was not accompanied by any practical application of the findings, and the plan for public works hardly got underway. In 1914 the Conservative government of Eduardo Dato (with Javier Ugarte as Minister of Development, a position he also held in later Liberal cabinets led by Count Romanones) launched measures to improve water supplies under the Public Water Works Act, which had been drawn up by the Liberal Minister Rafael Gasset in July 1911. They included the provision of a credit line to municipal governments for this purpose and the requirement for technical and medical expertise to be applied to the design and implementation of water supply projects. The introduction to the 1914 Decree acknowledged the role of the information collected by the RHB. However, these efforts failed, and the same orders had to be re-issued in November 1920 after an unsuccessful attempt to legislate on the issue.[34]

Malaria did not become a matter of national concern until 1920, when the Central Commission for the Sanitation of Malaria Regions was created.[35] This title owed more to the tradition of earth-borne diseases and environmental interventions represented by the RHB than to the activities of the bureau, since its

---

33 Data from 'Sanidad del Campo. Organización y servicios'. *Bol. Agric. Tec. Econ.* 1917; [July] nº 103: 614; 617-618, and Inspección de Sanidad del Campo. *Avances de los inventarios de Paludismo y Aguas Potables. Datos remitidos por los Inspectores Regionales.* Madrid: Ministerio de Fomento. Dirección General de Agricultura, Minas y Montes; 1918, 21.

34 RR.OO (Mº Fomento), *Gaceta* Jun 4 1914; March 1 1915; Nov 17 1920. 'Anteproyecto de ley de obras de abastecimiento y prestación de aguas potables…'. *Bol. Agric. Tecn. Econ.*, nº 84, (Dec 1915), 1004-1012.

35 Rodríguez-Ocaña, E; Ballester-Añón, R.; Perdiguero, E.; Medina-Doménech, R.M.; Molero, J. *La acción médico-social contra el paludismo en la España metropolitana y colonial del siglo XX*, Madrid, CSIC, 2003.

President, Pittaluga, adopted a far more human-oriented approach.[36] He considered 'major sanitation works' to be less important than the medical management of affected individuals, peri-domestic sanitation and the avoidance of contact with mosquitoes. Years earlier, the regional government of Catalonia had implemented the first modest official campaign against malaria, which served to establish a complete health department (1915-1924).[37] Although we cannot know the degree to which this initiative was influenced by the RHB surveys, they certainly added to the various political (nationalistic) and scientific pressures on the Catalonian authorities. Some local initiatives may also have resulted from the actions of regional officers and at least two of these, Colmenares in Valencia, and Suárez de Figueroa in Catalonia, published articles on the problem of drinking water in the local press.[38] Miguel Trallero, the Provincial Health Officer of Barcelona (under the Home Affairs Department), also carried out studies on this issue, always including a bacteriological analysis of the water.[39]

The RHB data on malaria were widely known and discussed. They were used by P. Hauser in his *Topografía Médica de la Península Ibérica* (1913) (Medical Geography of the Iberian Peninsula) and by Membrillera and Muñoz Antuñano, authors awarded prizes by the *Instituto de Ingenieros Civiles* (Civil Engineering Association) in 1921 for papers on 'the public health problem of Spain'.[40] The information also served as a rhetorical weapon for García Faria and others at the Spanish Public Health Association (*Sociedad Española de Higiene*) for the

---

36 Rodríguez-Ocaña, E.; Borowy, I. 'Gustavo Pittaluga (1876 – 1956). Science as a Weapon for Social Reform in a Time of Crisis', in Borowy, I. & Hardy, A. (eds.) *Of Medicine and Men. Biographies and Ideas in European Social Medicine between the World Wars*. Frankfurt a.M., Peter Lang, 2008, 173-196; Rodríguez-Ocaña, E.: 'International Health Goals and Social Reform: The Fight against Malaria in Interwar Spain', in Borowy, I. & Gruner, W.D. (eds.) *Facing Illness in Troubled Times. Health in Europe in the Interwar Years, 1918-1939*, Frankfurt a.M., Peter Lang, 2005, 247-276; Rodríguez-Ocaña, E. 'The birth of the anti-malaria campaign in Spain during the first 30 years of the 20th century: scientific and social aspects', *Parassitologia* 47 (2005), 371-377.

37 Bernabeu-Mestre, J. 'Cultura, ciencia y política. La lucha antipalúdica de la Cataluña de la Mancomunidad, 1914-1925', *Medicina e Historia*, nº 73 (1997).

38 Colmenares, I.G. 'El problema del agua potable'. *Policlínica*, 1916 (included among the printed sources of Barona, J.L. *Salud, enfermedad y muerte. La sociedad valenciana entre 1833 y 1939*, Valencia, Institució Alfons el Magnànim, 2002); Suárez de Figueroa, J. 'Las aguas potables en Cataluña. Avance de datos estadísticos de las aguas potables del partido judicial de Viella (provincia de Lérida)'. *Gac. Med. Catal.*, nº 953 (March 15 1917), 178.

39 Trallero, M. 'Las aguas en la provincia de Barcelona. Arenys de Mar'. *Gac. Med. Catal.*, 1915/2, 322-325; Badalona, *ibid.*, 365-373; Berga, Gac. *Med. Catal.*, 1916/1, p. 17-22; Calella, *ibid.*, 62-65; Manresa, *ibid.*, 99-102; Sitges, *ibid.*, 139-141.

40 G. de Membrillera, F. *El problema sanitario de España*, Barcelona, J. Viñals, 1921; Muñoz, L. *Saneamiento e higienización de España*, Madrid, Suc. Rivadeneyra, 1921.

commencement of a national anti-malaria campaign,[41] although Pittaluga's textbook *Enfermedades de los países cálidos y parasitología general* (Diseases of warm climates and general parasitology), questioned some of the data.[42]

Overall, RHB activities were restricted by the amount of data-gathering, the difficulties involved in this process, and by their limited capacity to correct data. Furthermore, the Bureau depended upon the activity of its regional officers, which varied according to the individual in question, and none were previously known in the public health sphere. They were also hampered by the usual deficiencies of the Spanish public administration of the time. Travel outside the locality of the assigned farm-school had to be approved and paid for by the central authority. The General Officer was supposed to decide about the number and exact date of travel days for every regional officer, according to both the 1913 and 1916 internal regulations, thus making inspection tours an uncommon event, as later recognised and criticised by a Rockefeller representative in 1925.[43] It was hard to conceive an effective work if officials in charge of environmental problems on a regional basis had to undergo a seemingly long bureaucratic procedure in Madrid in order to obtain permission to travel every time. Leaves of absence were also frequent, since the career of physicians at that time involved the gaining of one or more official positions simply to enhance their prestige. Several of the original officers resigned soon after their appointment, and the publication of regulations in 1916 concerning substitutions suggests this was a common occurrence.[44] And very important, there was also no linkage between the RHB and the public health structure with the exception of the General Officer, who sat on the Royal Health Board, the main advisory body. There were no connections at regional level, because the structure of national public health administration was based on the nation, the province and the municipality. It would evidently have been difficult for regional inspectors to establish meaningful working relationships with the numerous provincial and municipal health boards in their district.

---

41 García Faria, P. 'Lucha contra el paludismo. Discurso pronunciado en la Sociedad española de Higiene'. *Revista de Obras Públicas*, 68, nº 2361 (1920), 611-614. Others speakers were José Francos and Gustavo Pittaluga.

42 Pittaluga, G. *Enfermedades de los países cálidos y parasitología general*, Madrid, Calpe, 1923; 414 (Lerida) and 426 (Motril and nearby towns).

43 Rodríguez-Ocaña, E. '*El Informe sobre la sanidad española* (1926) de Charles A. Bailey, enviado de la Fundación Rockefeller', *Cronos*; 4 (2001), 63-79.

44 Officers from Old Castille, and the Balearic and Canary islands, resigned between 1911 and 1914. The Officer from Eastern Andalousia died in 1917, as did the one from Catalonia in early 1918.

The political framework of the Rural Health Bureau and its heritage

At the beginning of the twentieth century there were four urban views of the countryside that were not necessarily mutually exclusive: as an asset for economic growth; as a specific cultural area, characterised by poverty and tradition; as an aesthetic experience, reflected in art; and as a potentially dangerous place for living, thanks both to human agency (poor living and working conditions) and natural hazards, including mosquitoes and earth-borne diseases. In the domain of public health, this emerging consciousness of rural health risks, in combination with the idea of national regeneration, produced novel interventions at a time of scientific changes from the new disciplines of bacteriology and parasitology.

With the war against the USA lost in 1898, regeneration became the watchword in Spanish public discourse about the state and the future of the nation. The poor health data from Spain in comparison with European countries such as Germany, France or England increased frustrations. In the Liberal way of thinking, health problems were essentially about money and were considered in terms of their effects on the national economy, providing a rationale for investments in prophylactic measures. Notions of citizenship were only later added to this monetary reasoning, after the political dimension of rural distress became visible in riots and strikes, which reached their peak at the time of World War One.[45]

Although industry was the main target for development, an increase in land productivity also became an attractive goal after a growth in international earnings for some Spanish agricultural products, thanks to new trade networks and improvements in farming methods and transport. The desire for greater economic development led governments to extend their interests to rural areas at the beginning of the twentieth century, with a spate of data-gathering by the Commission and Institute for Social Reform.[46] Contributions from civil engineers were also outstanding, as they became the main professional force to sustain sanitation for the population, including hygienic dwellings, and water provision for drinking and for irrigation.[47] The Rural Health Bureau fitted perfectly this general trend in Spanish politics with regard to the peasant population, focusing

45 Rodríguez-Ocaña, 'Medicine as a Social Political Science'.

46 Viz. in 1900, 1902, 1903, 1906, 1919, 1920 and 1923. García Delgado, José L.; Sánchez Jiménez, J.; Tuñón de Lara, M. 'Los comienzos del siglo XX. La población, la economía, la sociedad', *Historia de España*, fundada por R. Menéndez Pidal, XXXVII, Madrid, Espasa Calpe, S.A., 1984; 308.

47 An approach to the role of civil engineering in rural health reforms is Galiana, Bernabeu-Mestre, 'El problema sanitario'.

on studies rather than reformist legislation or the implementation of truly effective interventions, and providing a medical legitimacy to public works.[48]

The first surveys of rural wages and life conditions of landless peasants in Andalucía and Extremadura were launched at the same time as the first National Irrigation Plan in 1902.[49] The so-called 'hydraulic policy' proved to be among the most long-lasting inheritances of the regenerationist movement, surviving under the military dictatorship of the 1920s and even inspiring Republican and Francoist public work programmes. The term was coined by Rafael Gasset (1866-1927), who was Minister of Development several times and owned *El Imparcial,* one of the main newspapers of the time.[50] The hydraulic policy was designed to upgrade agriculture by a combination of irrigation works and improved transportation, with the construction of local roads and railway lines. Gasset devised the programme, which was perfectly in line with the Engineering Association's policy of basing public works on technical information and not, as had been the rule, on the political influence of one or other member of the parliament. The setting up of the RHB meant that these public works would also be given a public health rationale, supporting a comprehensive approach to environmental health. This policy was not only followed by Liberal cabinets (under Canalejas, Moret or Count Romanones) but also by Dato's Conservative faction until the arrival of General Primo de Rivera in 1923.

The RHB was brought to an end by the Conservative government of Antonio Maura, known to be hostile to Gasset's policies.[51] As an organisation outside the official public health administration, it antagonised most physicians in this field. Public health, which came under the Ministry of Home Affairs, had a tradition of fighting epidemics and establishing pro-health regulations, one upheld by the staff which was campaigning for specialist training around the National Hygiene Institute created in 1899. None of this was considered in the selection of rural health officers, who were placed in a distinct administrative framework,

---

48 García Delgado, Sánchez Jiménez, Tuñón de Lara, 'Los comienzos del siglo XX', 310.

49 Malefakis, E. *Reforma agraria y revolución campesina en la España del siglo XX.* Barcelona, Ariel, 1972, 490. Monclús, F. J.; Oyón, J. L. *Historia y Evolución de la Colonización Agraria en España. I. Políticas y técnicas en la ordenación del espacio rural*, Madrid, Ministerio de Agricultura, Pesca y Alimentación, 1988, 81.

50 Gasset had first worked with the Conservatives but changed sides after the death of his close friend, Raimundo Fernández Villaverde (1848-1905). See Villanueva Larraya, G. 'Rafael Gasset: "La política hidráulica" en la acción del gobierno', *Rev Fac Geogr. Hist*, nº 1 (1987), 439-459; Sánchez Illán, Juan Carlos, 'Rafael Gasset y la política hidráulica de la Restauración, 1900-1923', *Rev. Hist. Econom.*, 15 (1997), 319-362.

51 Varela Ortega, J.; Dardé Morales, C. 'El movimiento regeneracionista y la crítica del sistema político de la Restauración'. In M. Espadas Burgos, coord. *La Época de la Restauración (1875-1902). Estado, política e islas de Ultramar*, Madrid, Espasa Calpe [*Historia de España de R. Menéndez Pidal*, XXXVI-1], 2000, 537-553.

despite political prescriptions for collaboration among different bodies of the administration.[52] However, the incipient state of the training facilities did not have to be a historical obstacle to the strengthening of the public health specialty, as demonstrated by the high success rate of the data-gathering activity. The main public health administration did not have a very distinguished record in this respect and resented unfavourable comparisons with another organisation in this area.[53]

Most public health campaigns started under private or mixed sponsorship, becoming incorporated into the National Health Department during the first third of the twentieth century. However, this was not the fate of the RHB. It was closed down and staff members were not offered alternative posts in public administration. The refusal of the public health sector to recognise the work of the Rural Health Officers has even tainted the historiography, in which the RHB is deemed a purely bureaucratic deviation from the trend towards truly scientific public health. It is true that the theory of earth-borne disease that framed the RHB was being undermined by microbiology and parasitology. However, if the two administrative bodies had been merged, a comprehensive public health approach could have been developed. Thus the RHB is a further illustration of the meetings between health problems and national strategies that gave birth to social medicine. It had some direct and indirect beneficial effects on the well-being of Spaniards, and its shortcomings can be better understood as a consequence of the general political and administrative situation.

52 RR.OO M° Gobernación. *Gaceta*, Jul 30 1911, 327; M° Fomento. *Gaceta*, Jun 6 1912, 551-552 and Feb 7 1914, 336. Circular order of the Dirección general de Agricultura, Minas y Montes. *Gaceta*, Jan 29 1916, 227.

53 During the existence of the RHB, the national health administration attempted unsuccessfully to produce a massive health survey in rural areas: RO, Gobernación. *Gaceta*, Jan 4 1911, 58.

SANITARY CAMPAIGNS AGAINST TRACHOMA IN RURAL SPAIN

Maria Eugenia Galiana, Ángela Cremades and Josep Bernabeu-Mestre

Throughout history, trachoma, the eye disease caused by the bacteria *Chlamydia trachomatis*, has been one of the major causes of 'avoidable' blindness. In the early twentieth trachoma was endemic in many parts of Europe. Papers presented to the 13th International Ophthalmological Congress, which took place in Amsterdam in 1929, underlined the incidence of the disease in Mediterranean countries and linked its recrudescence after World War One with the deterioration in living conditions experienced by large parts of the population.[1]

Spain was one of the European countries most affected, with an endemic area that extended all along its Mediterranean coast. Although the disease was declared notifiable by a Royal Decree dated January 10th 1919, [2] the first Spanish statistics on trachoma date back to 1924.[3] Interest in the trachoma endemic was particularly keen among the collective of ophthalmologists and expressed at the 13th Assembly of the Hispano-American Ophthalmological Society, held Seville in September 1923.[4] This agreed that trachoma as a condition should not provide grounds for exemption from military service and that the Society itself should constitute a national consultative centre for trachoma sufferers to attend. Indeed, the first statistics on trachoma came from the study carried out by two of the most reputed Spanish ophthalmologists of that era, Doctors Márquez and Soria. These indicated more than 45,000 trachoma sufferers and an incidence rate of 2.42 per 1,000 in the Spanish population, which, if anything, underestimated real levels.[5] As can be seen in Table 1, there were significant regional differences, with the highest incidence in the Mediterranean provinces of Murcia, Almería, Valencia, Castellón and Alicante.

1 Arjona y Trapote, J. and Alonso de Medina, F. *El tracoma*. Madrid, Aldecoa, 1941, 16-19.

2 Arjona y Trapote and Alonso de Medina, *El tracoma*, 136-137.

3 Ortíz de Landazuri, A. and Luengo, E. 'Spain', in *International Health Year-Book 1924*, Geneva, League of Nations. Health Organisations, 1925, 398-399.

4 López de Letona, C. 'La XIII Asamblea de la Sociedad Oftalmológica Hispano Americana (1923) y «el uso de los antojos» (1623)', *Arch Soc Esp Oftalmol.* (2006); 81: 49-50.

5 Alvarez Torres, R. *Algunas consideraciones sobre la profilaxis del tracoma en España*, Madrid, Publicaciones de Anales de la Beneficencia Municipal, 1927, 3.

Table 1. Trachoma distribution in Spain (by province), 1924

Province	Incidence per 1,000 inhabitants
Murcia	17.70
Almería	17.70
Valencia	12.78
Castellón	9.18
Alicante	3.36
Madrid	2.03
Zaragoza	2.03
Málaga, Logroño, Toledo, Tarragona, Palencia, Baleares, Albacete, Jaén	(between 1.82 Málaga and 1.05 Jaén).

Source: Ortíz de Landazuri, A. and Luengo, E. 'Spain', in *International Health Year-Book 1924*, Geneva, League of Nations Health Organisations, 1925, 398-399 (Statistics from the Márquez and Soria research).

This chapter considers the conceptual and methodological assumptions that informed the social struggle against trachoma in the 1920s and 1930s and analyses the prevalence of trachoma in rural areas. It utilises information brochures, monographs, articles and congress presentations published by the General Health Directory (*Dirección General de Sanidad*) or National Health Board (*Cuerpo Nacional de Sanidad*) staff responsible for the fight against trachoma.[6] It also draws upon papers by various ophthamologists, especially those who dealt with trachoma as a public health problem.[7]

Facing the problem in rural districts

The brochure published in 1915 by the Ministerio de la Gobernación (Ministry for Internal Affairs) represented the first national and institutionalised response to this disease. Introducing it, Doctor Martín Salazar, *Inspector General de Sanidad Exterior* (Inspector General for Foreign Health), condemned the delays and

6 Martín Salazar, M. *Lucha social contra el tracoma.* Madrid, Ministerio de la Gobernación. Publicaciones de las Inspecciones de Sanidad (serie monográfica), 1915; Alvarez Torres, R. *Algunas consideraciones.....*; Alvarez Torres, R. 'La lucha contra el tracoma en España', in: *Libro de Actas del Primer Congreso Nacional de Sanidad.* Madrid, Dirección General de Sanidad, 1934, 253-265; Jordano Barea, J. *Contribución al estudio de la extensión del tracoma en la provincia de Córdoba.* Córdoba, Instituto Provincial de Higiene, Sección de Oftalmología, 1935; Rabadán Fernández, P. 'Factores epidemiológicos en la zona tracomatosa de la provincia de Alicante'. *Revista de Sanidad e Higiene Pública* (1936), 416-422; Socias, A. and Delgado, J. 'Estudio de los factores epidémicos en la endemia tracomatosa'. *Revista de Sanidad e Higiene Pública* (1939), 1-47; Socias, A. 'Estudio de la distribución de la incidencia y de los factores epidémicos del tracoma en España, con un resumen de la distribución de la primera en todo el ecúmene'. *Revista de Sanidad e Higiene Pública* (1942), 371-403

7 Marín Amat, M. *Tracoma y sus complicaciones.* Madrid, Editorial Saturnino Calleja, 1923.

lack of resources needed to help control preventable diseases and explained the main objectives of the initiative.[8] One was to awaken curiosity and interest in studying trachoma, particularly amongst rural doctors: besides making a diagnosis and giving treatment, they needed to diffuse hygiene concepts amongst the population concerning its prevention and treatment.[9] With the assistance of the municipal and provincial health inspectors, this educational campaign could also compile data on the numbers affected.[10]

Specific measures involved the compulsory reporting of trachoma cases; the provision of free treatment; the systematic testing of all immigrants, particularly those from Portugal; and an educational campaign emphasising the importance of isolation of those affected to limit disease transmission.[11] However, the biggest challenge was to overcome the conditions that favoured the prevalence of trachoma, which thrived upon 'lack of cleanliness, of the presence of ignorance, poverty and of having poor people live in unhealthy housing'. This required fundamental improvements in the social and economic situation of the underprivileged classes. In much of the literature, trachoma was referred to as the 'poverty disease',[12] given the very poor living conditions that so much of the Spanish population had to contend with in the early twentieth century.[13] The situation in rural areas was particularly bad, with also some better off families living in unhealthy environments. Everywhere 'the armies of flies were a constant presence' and some of the poorest homes were cave dwellings, containing whole families and sometimes domestic animals. Some authors also commented upon 'an unforgivable messiness', suggesting that deficient personal habits were a contributory factor to the disease.[14] People rubbed their eyes, or picked out foreign bodies from the eyes with the hands or tongue, or resorted to eye washing with supposed 'miraculous waters': all noted by the health authorities as signs of ignorance, neglect and defective hygiene compounding a major problem. For Martín Salazar the worst consequence of trachoma as a social disease was that it prevented affected people from working and thereby intensified their poverty. As the 1915 pamphlet stated:

> 'When a man, in the best time of his life, at the time of his most physical and mental strength, finds himself invalidated for work because an illness has taken away his sight

---

8 Martín Salazar, *Lucha social*, 4-5.
9 Márquez, *La lucha contra el tracoma*, 11.
10 Martín Salazar, *Lucha social*, 5.
11 Martín Salazar, *Lucha social*, 12.
12 Rabadán, 'Factores', 416.
13 Galiana-Sánchez, M.E. and Bernabeu-Mestre, J. 'El problema sanitario de España: saneamiento y medio rural en los primeros decenios del siglo XX', *Asclepio*, 58(2) (2006), 139-164.
14 Arjona y Trapote and Alonso de Medina, *El tracoma*, 132.

> ... and when, due to ignorance or lazyness, the problem is passed on to other members of his own family ... then the picture of misery and poverty reaches the limits of unhappiness and misfortune. No one with a minimally sensitive heart can stand, without being shaken and without experiencing great pity, the sight of one of these poor, trachomose-ridden families, condemned to everlasting suffering and a deadly blindness.' [15]

Other problems centred upon the water cycle, for within high prevalence areas trachoma levels were noticeably lower where the necessary water supplies were available.[16]

However, the lack of rain in the most affected areas generally forced the population to limit water use severely. Where water was stored in cisterns its sanitary quality might be affected by proximity to septic tanks and to animal stables. There were also fewer possibilities of access to well water because underground water was at great depths and had a very high mineral content, which made it unusable for household, washing or farming purposes. Yet the situation was often no better where water was available from superficial or shallow wells as some of the worst morbidity occurred in areas taking water directly for domestic use or irrigation from rivers which had already passed through various towns and contained high levels of waste material.[17] Such water was usually simply stored in clay containers and traps with the aim of settling filth and sediments at the bottom. Moreover, some families lacked even clay pots or access to riverwater and were dependent upon collecting rainwater, often accumulated from roads or farmland, which might become very contaminated. In such circumstances hygiene habits were disastrously bad and the use of water for eye hygiene produced irritations of the conjunctiva and other repetitive infections. Thus many people with trachoma did not have the opportunity to carry out even a minimum of personal hygiene, so that secretions would build up in their conjunctiva, requiring health workers to separate their eyelashes with tweezers, a fraught and extremely painful process which provoked bleeding and made healing more difficult.

Another environmental factor that appeared to increase contagion by trachoma was settlement in areas in which the geological composition of the soil was rich in calcareous and saline constituents, accentuating the arid conditions. Coastal areas were particularly vulnerable, whereas mountainous areas were relatively free from contagion.[18] Epidemiological studies on trachoma also highlighted the subtropical climate of the affected areas, characterised by tempera-

---

15 Martín Salazar, *Lucha social*, 7-8.

16 Jordano, *Contribución*, 12.

17 Rabadán, 'Factores', 420.

18 Vila i Coro, A. *Tracoma. Aspecte mèdic i sanitari*. Barcelona, Monografies mèdiques (any VIII, núm. 75), 1933, 13; Socias, 'Estudio de la distribución de la incidencia…', 378-379.

tures exceeding 15° in the winter and reaching 50° in the summer, conditions which encourage microbiological proliferation, critical in the development of the disease. Furthermore, the diaphaneity of the environment frequently added to the effects of heat on the eyeball, imbuing solar radiation with maximum luminous intensity. Seasonal periodicity was also noted, the greatest number of cases occurring in the hottest months, from August to October. And, by carrying along large quantities of suspended matter, the intense winds present in some regions produced conjunctival erosion through mechanical action or toxicity through chemical action. The cumulative effect of these conditions was that the heat generated increased conjunctival oozing, altering the physical-chemical defence of the eyeball and encouraging the proliferation of germs. If more or less septic particulates, or particulates which could cause erosion, were deposited on the mucous membrane in these conditions, ideal conditions for trachomatous disease were created.[19]

Trachoma was clearly defined as a rural disease: filth, overcrowding, poverty and the lack of knowledge were considered the main features in its spread and so preventive individual and public hygiene measures were essential.[20] Individual recommendations varied from the complete isolation of all objects that were associated with the sick person's own hygiene, including clothes and bedclothing, the avoidance of personal contact such as handshaking and use of rigorous procedures of eye washing and disinfecting utensils. Trachoma sufferers were classified into those who could be cured because they followed hygiene habits and procedures, and those who were regarded as incurable because they had no knowledge or practice of hygiene.[21] The main public hygiene measures focused upon control of those affected to avoid disease transmission. The 1919 Royal Decree had proclaimed the compulsory declaration of all trachoma cases and, at the same time, ophthamologists' interest was increasing due to the social impact of this health problem. However, in the pamphlet published in 1925 by the *Dirección Nacional de Sanidad* [General Health Directorate], the influential ophthamologist Manuel Márquez insisted that trachoma was both preventable and curable, but that insufficient measures had been taken, and he denounced the lack of awareness and cooperation between health professionals and the authorities.[22]

However, the series of post-1927 health reforms put forward by the Primo de Rivera Dictatorship (1923-1931) began a systematic fight against trachoma with the establishment of a *Servicio Nacional Antitracomatoso* (National Anti-

19 Vila i Coro, *Tracoma*, 13-15.
20 Marín, *Tracoma*, 110-112.
21 Marín, *Tracoma*, 120.
22 Márquez, *La lucha contra el tracoma*, 5-7.

trachoma Service).[23] This initiative reflected both the institutionalisation of Spanish public health during the 1920s and 1930s and the cooperation agreement between Spain and the Rockefeller Foundation, which added an international health influence.[24] The Trachoma League was also established in Paris in 1927, followed by the League of Nations Health Committee International Organization Against Trachoma, which first met on July 26th 1930, and promoted specialist scientific publications, such as the *Revue Internationale du Trachome*. Dispensaries became the principal nucleus of anti-trachoma activity, boosting the role of health education.[25] As the secretary of the Comisión Central contra el Tracoma (Central Anti-Trachoma Committee), Doctor Alvarez Torres stated, the problem came down essentially to 'medical and social education'.[26] Medical education was necessary because of the need for the cooperation of health professionals in the diagnosis, declaration, treatment and follow-up care for those affected. Yet some doctors shielded themselves behind professional secrecy or feared that their patients would be stigmatised, which effectively hid trachoma cases from the specialists, making people 'run from them like from lepers'.[27] Social education was also needed to convince those affected that the disease was infectious with potentially serious consequences for the ill person and those in contact with him or her, particularly if the most elementary hygiene care was lacking or was not sustained to achieve a full recovery. The distribution of anti-trachoma dispensaries and specialised services, especially after the declaration of the Second Republic, reflected the geographic extension of the endemic and its intensity, as seen in Table 2.[28]

The primary dispensaries or local services, which were in the municipalities of the provinces most affected by trachoma, were responsible for sanitary vigilance and epidemiological control, but their main activity was the prophylaxis of individuals and families.[29] As trachoma affected the rural areas particularly, the preventive role of municipal health inspectors was very important. Normally the investigation and treatment process began with schools inspection and checks upon all the children in the municipality, who were gathered together by their school or local authorities. Ophthalmologists from the *Institutos Provinciales de Higiene* (Provincial Health Institutes) went to the various towns in vehicles that contained a small surgical space in order to carry out check-ups in the presence of the municipal health inspectors.

---

23 Alvarez, 'La lucha', 259.
24 Barona, J.L. and Bernabeu-Mestre, J. *La salud y el Estado. El movimiento sanitario internacional y la administración española (1851-1945)*, València, PUV, 2008, 231-262.
25 Jordano, *Contribución*, 14-18.
26 Alvárez, *Algunas*, 4.
27 Alvárez, *Algunas*, 4.
28 Alvárez, 'La lucha', 259; Arjona y Trapote and Alonso de Medina, *El tracoma*, 138-145.
29 Arjona y Trapote and Alonso de Medina, *El tracoma*, 138-139.

Table 2. Distribution by province of the anti-trachoma dispensaries and specialized services, Spain (1934)

Province	**Dispensaries**	**Specialised Services**	**Ophthalmology Clinics (Provincial Hospitals)**
Alicante	13	2	1
Murcia	13	2	
Almería	10	2	1
Granada	8		
Castellón	5	2	
Valencia	5	1	
Cádiz	4		
Cáceres	3		
Córdoba, Huelva, Jaén, Madrid and Malaga	2 each		
Badajoz, Huesca, Gran Canaria, Mellila and Toledo	1 each		

Source: Alvarez Torres, R. 'La lucha contra el tracoma en España', in *Libro de Actas del Primer Congreso Nacional de Sanidad*, Madrid, Dirección General de Sanidad, 1934, 253-265; Arjona y Trapote, J. and Alonso de Medina, F. *El tracoma*, Madrid, Aldecoa, 1941, 138-145.

When the list of trachoma patients was established, local doctors from each municipality and rural health centre followed up by making appointments for family members and other relations of the sick people for check-up and detection of possible new cases.[30] The process was completed by domiciliary inspections by the homecare and visiting nurses.[31] These professionals played an essential role, especially in the detection of new cases and in the 'pedagogical task of promoting hygienic guidelines' for, as one text put it, 'if sick people do not come, we have to go look for them'. It added, in relation to the homecare and visiting nurses, that 'It would be good if the State institutions and charity multiply the number of these selfless professionals, as we cannot forget that the first step of any health model is a perfect hygiene in the customs, person and home'.[32]

Trachoma prophylaxis began with the medical examination of pregnant women, who had been referred by ophthalmologists, and continued with health visitors, who sent other family members suffering from granular disease to the dispensaries, in particular women, who had most contact with the new-born, and ended with surveillance of the child's health in terms of food, hygiene and eye

30 Alvárez, *Algunas*, 4; Alvárez, 'La lucha'.

31 Jordano, *Contribución*, 16.

32 Arjona y Trapote and Alonso de Medina, *El tracoma*, 135.

care.[33] Ongoing health information, regular home visits, well-managed breast-feeding and appropriate treatment of diseases which could cause constitutional defects could, in the opinion of Spanish health practitioners, prevent 'the lack of cleanliness, promiscuity, lymphatism, avitaminosis, conjunctivitis neonatorum and many other factors which are so important in the aetiology of infection'. [34]

As indicated, Spanish health professionals considered that 'infectious diseases in general, hereditary defects or inadequate nutrition which produce physical decline' all predisposed people to trachoma and aggravated the disease. Thus Arjona and Alonso proposed:

> 'Increasing the lifestyle of the lower classes and fighting against everything which has been proved to produce organic poverty (alcoholism, tuberculosis, syphilis, overwork) … above all, breast-feeding will be closely observed and particularly bottle-feeding, where it must be ensured that the child is taking in sufficient levels of vitamins A and C, as these vitamins powerfully stimulate lysozyme concentration. This factor has the greatest effect on local receptivity, which is so important in the early years of life. From here also arises the need to fight against scrofula through vitamin and antitubercular therapy'.[35]

As the head of the anti-trachoma campaign, Doctor Alvárez noted that health education was always made difficult by the misery, poverty and ignorance of trachoma patients, which not only promoted disease transmission but also made prophylaxis and treatment that much harder. Health professionals rapidly identified their main obstacles as the 'lack of education, laziness and even certain superstitions', which resulted in sick people not attending medical clinics and thereby required further background educational work and even 'preaching'.[36] Underdevelopment and all prejudices against the dirty rural were explicit:

---

33 The head of the Trachoma Section of the Health Department defined the evolution of trachoma in the endemic zone of the Spanish Levante thus (Alvárez, 'La lucha', 255): 'In our area of the Levante, where trachoma is endemic, its clinical evolution could be said to start in early childhood – latent infection – from a trachoma hotspot or a contagion-producing medium and continues its silent march without complications until the child reaches school age or adolescence, when an outbreak of 'super-infection' occurs, which may be short or long-lasting, but which is always followed by a series of outbreaks, present in adults with differing frequency … in addition to this latent infection in childhood, we have cases of adolescent and adult contamination, which require intimacy and continuity of infective contact, and contagion is thus less frequent but easier, and individual prophylaxis has been shown to have more positive results … health efforts must consequently be focused on the child, especially while still breast-feeding, and in this respect Rural Health Centres are of great importance'.

34 Alvarez, 'La lucha', 255.

35 Arjona y Trapote and Alonso de Medina, *El tracoma*, 141.

36 Alvarez, 'La lucha', 253.

> 'The mentality of the farmworkers is that for them the diseases of the farm animals and transport animals are more important, that it affects them more economically than an eye problem that, although it can be a bother, when it does not have a lot of discharge, nor a lot of pain nor affects the eyesight greatly ... does not keep them from working. Because of this, instead of going ... for a treatment that, besides being painful, they consider unnecessary, they let the problem evolve and they transmit it to their family members until some complication forces the to go see the eye doctor – who generally lives in the provincial capital – and it is then that the lack of economic means motivate, perhaps because they have to be hospitalized or they stop the treatment as soon as they feel a bit better.' [37]

Given this situation, in addition to raising popular awareness of the seriousness of the problem, the health authorities involved insisted on the need to start with treatment for active or 'current' cases, whilst reserving the possibility of applying more coercive measures.[38]

Among the functions of the local services were school inspections and the treatment and follow-up of children with trachoma. However, the School Medical Inspectorate, created by Decree of April 17th 1933, assumed responsibility among its other functions for treating all trachoma cases and other contagious eye diseases, for investigation and treatment of the family members of affected children, and for providing them with the necessary understanding of 'hygiene and health'. Spanish health professionals continually reported that, for their interventions to be successful, trachoma treatment had to be obligatory. They also indicated that, 'instead of keeping trachoma sufferers away from schools, based on misunderstood isolation', these should be treated in annexed dispensaries, thus leading to the creation of special schools for trachoma sufferers, a project which had already been prepared but not yet put into practice.[39]

Another area which benefited from the prophylactic activity was workplace-related campaigning. Besides sea fishing, 'at-risk' activities included the esparto grass industry, tanning and ceramics.[40] The reaping tasks in farming were similarly hazardous as these were performed at the hottest time of the year and obliged workers to stay in the fields, exposing their eyes to irritations produced by dust from roads, soil, crops and fertilizers. Consequent corneal and conjuncti-

---

37 Alvarez, *Algunas*, 4-5.

38 Martín Salazar, *Lucha social*, 5; Márquez, *La lucha contra el tracoma*, 7.

39 Trachoma sufferers without secretions presented little danger to others if they observed hygiene rules. It was better for active trachoma sufferers to remain at school, since they could thus be treated and controlled. Kept away from school, not only were they condemned to illiteracy, but they also stopped attending dispensaries clinics and health services, thus becoming a source of contagion within the family and their wider circle and contributing to the spread of trachoma. See Alvárez, 'La lucha', 256-7.

40 Socias and Delgado, 'Estudio', 43-46.

val irritations, with their traumatic action, opened the way for infection. As one annual report published by the anti-trachoma dispensaries explained:

> 'In the esparto grass factories, the lack of hygiene and the poverty of the workers is added to the large amounts of dust, which is so great, especially in the departments in which the esparto grass is crushed. There, it is materially impossible to breathe and those who work there have their faces covered by the dust.'[41]

Similarly, rural migrations contributed to the spread and worsening of endemic trachoma, of particular significance in Barcelona city and many Catalan towns. As Vila i Coro's study acknowledged, large numbers of migrants came from very poor and trachoma-affected rural regions, such as Murcia, Almería, Alicante and Castellón, in search of work opportunities in Catalan industries.[42] With no *cordon sanitaire* and given the overcrowding and lack of hygiene in the poor accommodation where such groups lived, the situation was aggravated, turning Barcelona into one of the cities with the highest levels of trachoma in Spain. In 1927 it was calculated that the rate of trachoma infections in the city was 15 per 1,000 inhabitants, when in 1910 it had been barely one per 1,000. Whereas other countries had strict regulations to prevent trachoma sufferers from entering or which controlled their movement, Spanish legislation did not include such measures.[43] This explains the public health problems experienced in parts of French Algeria by groups of Spanish trachoma sufferers from the provinces of Alicante and Almería who temporarily emigrated there, with no controls exercised by the Spanish authorities.[44]

> 'In Spain there are no regulations to protect us from the importation of trachoma by foreigners, above all Moroccans, Hungarians, gypsies and individuals coming from Portugal and the south of France. Even within our own country, we have sufferers who travel (from trachoma zones to previously unaffected areas) in search of work, leading to real epidemics of granular ophthalmia.'[45]

Spanish health professionals also called for the creation of asylums to treat trachoma sufferers with no personal means of support, a measure evidently considered indispensable for a variety of reasons:

---

41 Alvarez, 'La lucha', 257.

42 Vila i Coro, *Tracoma*, 11-12.

43 Arjona y Trapote and Alonso de Medina, *El tracoma*, 145-151.

44 Arjona y Trapote and Alonso de Medina, *El tracoma*, 19. In the region of Oran, 66% of trachoma sufferers were of Spanish origin. This featured in a paper filed on the lack of control and its consequences, see Alvárez, 'La lucha', 258.

45 Alvarez, 'La lucha', 258.

> 'Trachoma being a disease which is almost always accompanied by abandonment, promiscuity and poverty ... beggars with granular disease and those blinded by trachoma, far from wandering the streets, should be rounded up and isolated in special centres, where they can receive appropriate treatment, while at the same time being removed from contact with the public, thus avoiding further contagion.'[46]

Conclusions

According to health professionals responsible for dealing with the trachoma problem in early twentieth-century Spain, the fundamental issue was a lack of personal and public hygiene, with the 'dirty rural' and peasants' rudeness cited as particular causes. Environmental features included the sub-tropical climate, which characterised the majority of rural endemic areas, along with the diaphaneity of the environment, the winds and aridity, as well as problems associated with the water cycle and scarcity, along with health risks in particular occupations.

Under health reforms and the modernisation of Spanish public health during the 1920s and early years of the Second Republic, anti-trachoma measures included prophylaxis, preventive and educational activities and the inspections carried out by the dispensaries and the rural health centres. Faced with some lack of cooperation from the population, it was fundamental that work undertaken by health professionals in the rural areas involved active searches and the early detection of cases, alongside efforts to modify those risk factors associated with unhygienic living conditions, work activities and popular habits. Ultimately, such measures contributed to the eradication of trachoma in Spain in the 1960s.[47] This serves to reaffirm the validity of such strategies in dealing with similar health problems in poorer areas of the world: improvements in the hygienic conditions and underlying environmental factors, through transversal community interventions, seem essential.[48]

---

46 Alvarez, 'La lucha', 259

47 Gimeno de Sande, A. *Memoria sobre la Campaña Nacional de Lucha contra el Tracoma*, Madrid, Ministerio de la Gobernación. Dirección General de Sanidad, 1964-1965.

48 Konyama, K. 'History of trachoma control in Asia', *Revue internationale du trachome et de pathologie oculaire tropicale et subtropicale et de santé publique*, 81-82 (2004-2005), 107-168.

POLIOMYELITIS IN RURAL AND URBAN SPAIN: EPIDEMIOLOGICAL TRENDS, SOCIAL AND SCIENTIFIC RESPONSES[1]

María José Báguena, María Isabel Porras and Rosa Ballester

This chapter analyses the Spanish experience of poliomyelitis and the distribution of mortality and morbidity rates according to environmental features and also to social and professional responses to this problem, both in rural and urban areas. The relationship between disease and environment and the contrast between the development of infectious diseases in town and countryside are not new subjects in historiography.[2] Most studies on the history of twentieth-century poliomyelitis outbreaks have noted the fundamental role of environmental factors such as climate and seasons of the year, social and sanitary conditions and, more specifically, of urban and rural settings. For example, the distribution of polio cases in Western countries showed that the disease affected both towns and countryside, although its incidence could vary between slums and districts with better social and sanitary conditions within the same town. The distribution of morbidity and mortality by age, social class and severity of the disease, also differed among rural, suburban and city areas, and changes in local circumstances within an area during the twentieth century influenced the incidence and distri-bution of the disease.

These general features have been well established in historical studies on polio in several Western countries.[3] From the 1920s onwards, epidemiological

---

1 This work is part of the Project 'La Poliomielitis en la España del siglo XX: repercusiones científicas, profesionales y sociales', financed by the Science and Education Ministry (HUM2005-07378-C03-01/HIST; HUM2005-07378-C03-02/HIST).

2 Hannaway, C. 'Environment and miasmata', in Bynum, W.F. and Porter, R. (eds.) *Companion Encyclopedia of the History of Medicine*, London, Routledge, 1993, 292-308; Porter, R. 'Diseases of Civilization', in Bynum and Porter, 'Companion', 585-600; Kippel, K.F. 'The ecology of disease', in Bynum and Porter, 'Companion', 357-381; Berridge, V. 'From environmentalism to personal prevention', in *Health and Society in Britain since 1939*, Cambridge, Cambridge U.P., 1999, 48-54; Mitman, G.; Murphy, M.; Sellers, C. (eds.) 'Landscapes of exposure: knowledge and illness in modern environments', *Osiris* (second series), 19 (2004).

3 For papers centred on the USA, see Wilson, D. 'A crippling fear: experiencing polio in the era of FDR', *Bulletin of History of Medicine*, 72 (1988), 464-495; Rogers, N. *Dirt and Disease. Polio before FDR*, New Brunswick, Rutgers U.P., 1992; Gould, T. *A summer plague: polio and its survivors*, New Haven/ London, Yale University Press, 1995; Black, K. *In the shadow of Polio: a personal and social history*, Reading, Addison-Wesley, 1996; Sass, E. *Polio's legacy. An oral history*, Lanhan, London, University Press of America,

studies analysed when and how polio affected human populations and the introduction of serological surveys in the 1950s added new information on the immunological status of communities. These main sources allow us to delineate three stages in the development of polio in relation to urban and rural variables in Western countries. First, around 1900 there were no differences between rural and urban areas and polio was associated with the poorest, dirtiest children; non-affluent adults in the prime of life and, in countries such as the USA, with immigrants in slum districts.[4] However, from the 1920s and 1930s a new image of polio arose as a disease of cleanliness, especially relevant in the great epidemics of the 1940s and 1950s, which centred upon the towns, with urban children from middle and higher social classes more likely to be affected than children who lived in slums. Third, after 1955, with the widespread use of vaccination with inactivated poliovaccine (IPV) and attenuated oral poliovaccine (OPV), the number of cases fell dramatically in the 1960s and 1970s. As not all children were immunised, small epidemics still occurred among the poor living in substandard conditions, whether urban or rural.

The transformation of the relatively uncommon 'infantile paralysis' of the nineteenth century into the almost worldwide 'poliomyelitis epidemic', was one of the most formidable twentieth century public health problems in Spain as in other Western countries.[5] The prevailing current explanation regarding the

---

1996; Shell, M. *Polio and its aftermath. The paralysis of culture*, Cambridge, Harvard U.P., 2005; Oshinsky, D.M. *Polio. An American story*, Oxford, Oxford U.P., 2005. There is less information on Europe but see: Lindner, U. and Blume, S. 'Vaccine innovation and adoption: polio vaccines in the UK, the Netherlands and West Germany, 1955-1965', *Medical History, 50* (2006), 425-446. Other British examples include: Webster, Ch. *The Health Services since the War: Volume II. Government and Health Care. The National Health Service 1958–1979*, London, HMSO, 1996, 129-131; Rogers, N. 'Silence has its own Stories: Elizabeth Kenny, Polio and the Culture of Medicine', *Social History of Medicine*, 21(2008), 145-161. A much-cited classic study is Paul, J.R. *A History of Poliomyelitis*, New Haven/London, Yale U.P., 1971.

4 Rogers '*Dirt and Disease*'.

5 For Spain see: Báguena Cervellera, M.J. 'Saberes y prácticas en torno a la polio en la medicina valenciana (1900-1950)', in Martínez Pérez, J.; Porras Gallo, M.I.; Samblas Tilve, P.; Del Cura González, M. (eds.) *La Medicina en el nuevo milenio. Una perspectiva histórica*, Cuenca, Ed. UCLM, 2004, 949-962; Martínez Navarro, F. et al. 'Estudio de la epidemia de poliomielitis infantil presentada en Madrid durante el año 1929 por el Dr. Laureano Albadalejo. Primera memoria anual de los trabajos llevados a cabo por el Servicio Epidemiológico Central (1929)', in Martínez; Porras; Samblas Tilve; Del Cura, 'La Medicina', 963-987. Ballester, R. 'Isabel Morgan y el grupo de investigación sobre vacunas de la Universidad Johns Hopkins (1940-1960): un modelo de análisis de la trayectoria de una mujer en el mundo de la ciencia', *Feminismos, 10* (2007), 119-135. Ballester, R. 'La presentación internacional de las campañas de vacunación contra la poliomielitis en España', in Perdiguero Gil, E. *Las vacunas. Historia y actualidad*, Menorca, Institut d'Estudis Menorquins, 2008, 123-138.

transformation of polio from an uncommon illness to a feared epidemic disease emphasises the importance of improvements in hygiene and sanitation. As noted in Per Axelsson's consideration of the Swedish case, a simplistic explanation is often used to illustrate the epidemic development of polio. [6] Until the late nineteenth century, all infants were exposed to the common virus but maternal antibodies that led to lifelong immunity against polio protected them. However, sanitation improvements in many western countries provided a healthier environment and made the virus less common. Consequently fewer infants were exposed to it, which then raised the proportion of unexposed individuals susceptible to polio later in life. Moreover, hygiene improvements were most often initiated in urban areas with relatively high living standards, which made the higher and middle social classes most susceptible to the virus. For this reason polio was considered a disease caused by civilisation and increased the feeling of fear among these groups of population.

Urban development and population concentration raise questions concerning illness and its social repercussions. [7] First, the concentration of people in a reduced space increases health risks and enhances the spread of epidemics precisely by increasing the possibility of contagion. Second, the health problems of citizens have generated various social responses and have acted as an impulse to scientific developments, public health practices, and the foundation of care institutions and of innovative organisational models. Finally, since the phenomenon of urban growth, understood as a process, also implies changes in the behaviour of town dwellers, then towns are places where intellectual forums, environments and spaces for reflection arise and the phenomenon of associations flourishes.

In the case of polio, the relationship between town and disease had specific characteristics. From 1950 onwards polio was seen as a setback for the welfare state and sanitary reforms. In 1950 Sven Gard explained the epidemiology of polio in terms of population density, climate and general levels of hygiene, setting out the new theory on the origins of the disease for the first time.[8] He supported the oral-faecal means of contagion and thus insisted that polio must have existed since prehistoric times: the symbiosis between germs and host had developed over thousands of years and was made possible by an unhygienic way of life. However, the adoption of hygiene measures changed the balance between virus and host. Polio was thus an environmental disease, the price to pay for sanitary improvements which had helped to control the plague, cholera and

---

6 Axelsson, P. *Hostens spöke. De svenska polioepidermias historia*, Stockolm, Carlssons, 2004 [with a summary in English, 230-238].

7 Valero Lobo, A. 'El sistema urbano español a lo largo del siglo XX', in Gonzálvez Pérez, V. *Los procesos de urbanización: siglos XIX y XX*, Alicante, Instituto de Cultura 'Juan Gil Albert', 1991, 9-23.

8 Gard, S. 'Problem of poliomyelitis virus', *Revue Neurologique, 83* (1) (1950), 29-30.

other epidemic fevers, and definitively a 'disease of civilisation'.[9] For this reason it had survived improvements in sanitary conditions in western cities and civilisation was thus a contributor to polio as a serious health problem. Gard's hypothesis stimulated further research into the distribution of polio by age group and urban or rural areas. Thus the age of contagion was higher in developed than poorer countries, as contact with the virus occurred later as a result of the sanitary reforms. This was even more obvious in isolated rural areas where the possibilities of exposure to the virus were fewer than in the towns.

There was also an important international movement against polio epidemics headed by the World Health Organisation and reports of the Expert Committee on Poliomyelitis from 1953 onwards related environmental factors to immunity. Already in the 1940s, America's medical research community had generally accepted the view of poliomyelitis as an intestinal viral infection, which implied the mouth as route of entry and faecal contamination as the means of transmission. Poor sanitary conditions and contamination of the environment thus favoured the spread of the disease. Given the new prevailing paradigm, there was a re-evaluation of roles played by climate, the seasons of the year, flies, hygienic and sanitary conditions, poverty, and population density. Environmental factors acquired renewed importance and the application of modern studies of immunity, begun in the 1930s, encouraged their acceptance by the scientific community. The WHO Expert Committee presented reports in 1954, 1956, 1958 and 1960, some of which established urban and rural differences in the acquisition of im-munity to polio. In urban populations, the acquisition of antibodies against the three different types of polio viruses seemingly took place at approximately the same age whereas, in rural and isolated communities, the times at which the re-spective viruses appear in the community might not necessarily be identical and might occur in successive waves.

In accordance with the dominant theories on the aetiology of polio the outbreaks in Spain in the 1940s and 1950s meant, from the perspective of Spanish health authorities, the alignment of an impoverished country, whose international prestige had been damaged by its political regime, with the rest of the 'civilised' nations.[10] The result was that authorities focussed upon the fight against polio especially in urban surroundings, although the beginning of this fight can be traced to the 1920s. In Spain poliomyelitis morbidity and mortality rates increased during the 1950s until the end of 1963, when the massive poliomyelitis vaccination campaign was launched. This increase was evident at national level and in the three main cities, Madrid, Barcelona and Valencia. The

9 Porter, 'Diseases of Civilization'.

10 Ballester, R. and Porras, M.I. 'Child protection as a political resource: the influence of international agency advice on sanitary campaigns against poliomyelitis in Spain'. Unpublished paper.

Spanish morbidity rate peaked in 1959 at 7.12 per 100,000 inhabitants and rates in the provinces of Madrid, Barcelona and Valencia were above the national average, at 8.68, 19.02 and 8.94 respectively.[11] In the province of Barcelona, morbidity rates decreased before a new peak of 5.10 in 1963 and similarly in the province of Valencia, (6.08 in 1963), but still below 1959 levels. However, morbidity levels for the province of Madrid continued to rise until 1963, the peak of 19.68 higher even than in 1959.[12]

Spain's battle with polio had several fronts. The government created polio health services, including special wards in hospitals, a national network of iron lungs and, above all, mass vaccination campaigns, using the problem of polio as a propaganda tool both inside the country and abroad. Indeed, the showcasing of these achievements in forums such as the European Conferences on Polio was a major part of the Spanish authorities' efforts to secure some form of international legitimisation of the political regime. Yet that was only part of the story. Contributions were also made by the voluntary sector and other self-help initiatives, although these were less frequent than in other Western countries. They included a Spanish Society against Polio and a series of leaflets containing self-help advice for the care of polio sufferers at home. Catholic religious congregations also provided care for children with disabilities – polio patients included – in special institutions throughout Spain. Finally, polio occasioned fundamental field trials for more or less orthodox therapies, in some cases the last hope for polio victims.

The fight against poliomyelitis in Spain can be divided into three stages: the emergence of polio from the 1890s; the outbreaks of the 1940s and 1950s; and pathways to the polio vaccination campaign in the 1960s. Each had its specific characteristics and all have a bearing upon rural-urban issues because of the changing distribution of polio morbidity and mortality rates during the period studied. Differences in the development of strategies of health intervention also emerged, with therapeutic resources for acute stage poliomyelitis increasingly likely to be located in towns, whereas preventive measures, especially the massive vaccination campaign of 1963-64, were widespread as authorities sought to protect all Spanish children from polio and major efforts indeed targeted inhabitants of the most isolated rural areas.

---

11 The provinces encompass rural and urban populations, excluding provincial capitals, with morbidity and mortality statistics for each capital and province, but not for respective rural areas. In the cities in 1959 there were 154 cases of polio in Madrid, 297 in Barcelona and 32 in Valencia.

12 There were 32 cases in Valencia city in 1961 and 29 in 1963; with 86 in 1961 and 88 in 1963 in the city of Barcelona. For Madrid itself there were 281 cases in 1961, 354 in 1962 and 510 in 1963. Data from the Statistics National Institute within the General Health Department and Nájera, E. et al. 'Análisis epidemiológico de la situación actual de la poliomielitis en España', *Revista de Sanidad e Higiene Pública, 49* (1975), 953-1025.

Polio in Spain 1890s-1930s

Sporadic manifestations of poliomyelitis in late nineteenth-century Spain gave rise to the first medical publications and activities on the disease, with a wide variety of treatments, the majority of which were criticised for their lack of verified efficacy.[13] At least three types of obstacles existed. First, it was difficult to make an early diagnosis of infantile paralysis since the initial symptoms were so unspecific and common to almost all infectious illnesses. Second, the variety of clinical forms and the different types of virus meant that the accumulated experience from one epidemic could not be applied to another and, third, the evolution of the disease was unpredictable: sometimes the paralysis was overcome without any treatment. The fundamental aims were to reduce mortality, to treat symptoms and to ensure that the subsequent disability was minimised.

Poliomyelitis became a prominent medico-social problem in the first half of the twentieth century, acquiring greater visibility with isolated outbreaks before the Civil War. Although the works of the Swedish paediatrician Ivar Wickman aroused immediate interest among Spanish doctors, it was not until the 1910s that it was possible to see a clearer influence of the ideas set out by Wickman, Simon Flexner or Wade Hampton Frost, among others. The first survey in Spain, designed by the Professor of paediatrics, Ramón Gómez Ferrer, was presented to the third Spanish Congress of Obstetrics, Gynaecology and Paediatrics in 1913.[14] It included the scientific background and debate on the entry route (respiratory or digestive) of the polio virus and results of the survey of the Valencia region. Ferrer noted the increased incidence of polio, especially in rural villages and among children under three years of age. He urged the Government to introduce obligatory notification of cases of poliomyelitis, reflecting general concerns over this and other infectious diseases, at the time seen as 'avoidable diseases'.[15]

---

13 'The experience shows that the worse the results are, the greater the number of treatments proposed', Suárez de Puga, L.'Poliomielitis. Segunda parte de estudio crítico de los tratamientos de la páralisis infantil', *Acta Pediátrica Española*, 43 (1946), 961-2.

14 Gómez Ferrer, R. 'Parálisis espinal infantil. Etiología y patogenia', in *Actas III Congreso español de Obstetricia, Ginecología y Pediatría*, Valencia, 1913, 299-331.

15 The term 'avoidable' is applied to those infectious illnesses which medical science had discovered 'safe ways of preventing'. Martín Salazar, M. *La Sanidad en España. Discurso de ingreso en la Real Academia de Medicina*, Madrid, Imprenta del Colegio Nacional de Sordomudos y de Ciegos, 1913, 51, 53.

With its parliamentary political system in crisis, Spain was in the midst of serious social, political and economic upheaval, with doctors and hygienists drawing attention to the backwardness of the country in health terms and the need for thoroughgoing reform and modernisation of the health system. Reacting to the great epidemic in New York in 1916, the Inspector General of Health decided to undertake a 'health campaign against infantile paralysis in Spain', requesting the Royal Academy of Medicine to include poliomyelitis, an 'avoidable disease', among the notifiable diseases.[16] While doctors did little to comply with this obligation, polio did receive greater attention, as seen in the 1917 epidemic in Barcelona.[17] Yet there was no epidemiological research until the 1920s, reflecting health reforms prompted by renewed debate concerning health care in Spain during the influenza pandemic of 1918-1919.

With a further epidemic of poliomyelitis in Madrid in 1929, the Central Epidemiological Service, an institution created during the dictatorship of Primo de Rivera, took responsibility for carrying out this research.[18] It utilised comprehensive epidemiological files on the hygienic and sanitary situation of the patients, human contact with insects to test existing theories concerning poliomyelitis transmission and also featured careful analysis of the geographical and age distribution of cases. [19] The latter revealed that 91 per cent of cases occurred in children aged under five years and 99.5 per cent in those younger than 15 years, although urban-rural differences were not discernible.

The most important therapeutic measures involved the introduction of serotherapy and the initial use of the hospital. Some Spanish doctors considered that an important tool in the acute stage of poliomyelitis was convalescent serum, as Arnold Netter had shown, and additional treatments – chemical, physical and electrical – were proposed.[20] The newly opened National Hospital for Infectious Diseases (*Hospital del Rey*) had a special polio ward and its director, Manuel Tapia, used convalescent serum solely or in combination with diathermy, electrotherapy and deep radiotherapy, following Bordier's method, with some 112

16 This approach signalled a national fight against the poliomyelitis in Spain.

17 Viura y Carreras, J. 'La parálisis infantil y su propagación en Cataluña', *Anales de la Real Academia de Medicina y Cirugía de Barcelona*, 1917, 1-17.

18 Albaladejo, L. 'Estudio de la epidemia de poliomielitis infantil presentada en Madrid durante los cuatro últimos meses del año 1929'. In Servicio epidemiólogico central. *Primera memoria anual de los trabajos llevados a cabo por el Servicio Central. Año 1929.* Madrid, Ministerio de la Gobernación, 1930, 106-159.

19 The poliomyelitis case distribution in Madrid was: capital (67%); province (21%); rural places and others receiving care in Madrid (12%).

20 Martín Salazar, 'La Sanidad', 19-22; Viura, 'La parálisis infantil', 15-16; Garrido Lestache, J. *Tratamiento de la poliomielitis anterior aguda o parálisis espinal infantil.* Madrid, Impr. de Cándido Alonso, 1915. See also Bastos Ansart, M. *Tratamiento de la parálisis infantil por el médico general.* Madrid, Edit. Saturnino Calleja, 1921.

patients.[21] The convalescent serum was provided by children of the *Asilo-Hospital de San Rafael* of Madrid (Hospital Order of Saint John of God), the most important religious institution caring for polio patients.[22]

In Valencia, the *Asilo Hospital de San Juan de Dios* opened at the Malvarrosa Beach in 1913, aiming as with all such centres to 'take in care for and treat children with tuberculosis, rachitis, ringworm, physical handicap and poor orphans'.[23] The Malvarrosa Beach, some three kilometres from the city centre, was the chosen location for several specialised hospitals for the treatment of skeletal diseases. Initially the clinic took care of children with skeletal tuberculosis and congenital or acquired disabilities requiring surgical-orthopaedic treatment, including those suffering the effects of infant paralysis. The difficulties involved were stated by Jorge Comín Vilar, the honorary director:

> 'There is a group of patients suffering the effects of infantile paralysis who deserve special medical-surgical treatment, and this led us to think of the advantages of transferring them to other centres belonging to the Order, to see if they could obtain better functional results than we had, as in the service there was a lack of ad hoc installations to achieve the pertinent muscle movement recovery.'[24]

Several surgical and orthopaedic treatments were performed on deformities and contractures attributed to a failure to use postural treatment during the period of regression of motor paralysis.[25] The most common operation at this time to treat a paralytic foot was the double tarsus arthrodesis.[26] Children unable to walk stayed in the Invalid Department, where there was a school and separate facilities, and were wheeled out onto terraces facing the sea in order to sun-bathe. When they were able to move, they attended morning and afternoon classes, their recovery completed with physical exercise on the patio and hospital

---

21 Tapia, M. 'Estudio clínico de la epidemia de poliomielitis de Madrid en 1929', *La Medicina Ibera*, 652 (1930), 621-628; 653, 657-663.

22 This institution was created in 1892 in Pinto (Madrid). It transferred to the city of Madrid around 1900, moving into a new building in 1914, acquiring great importance in the orthopaedic treatment of disabled children (scrofulosis, rachitis, infantile paralysis...). It also received children from rural areas.

23 Burguera Serrano, A. *Reseña histórico-descriptiva del Asilo de San Juan de Dios de Valencia*, Valencia, José Ortega, 1913, 8.

24 *ASILO hospital de San Juan de Dios. Memoria del año 1933*, Valencia, Imprenta Ortega, 1934, 51. That year five of the 93 in-patients suffered from infant parálisis and 76 operations were performed, 4 upon paralysed feet (ibid, 59-60).

25 'Asilo', 104-105.

26 'Asilo', 106. The head of the Infant Surgery and Orthopaedic Section was the Hospital manager, José Alvarez Santolino, the first specifically surgeon-paediatrician in Valencia.

grounds, with Swedish gymnastics, two walks a week and 'tónicos' baths in summer.[27]

Also located on Malvarrosa Beach was the *Asilo Hospital de Nuestra Señora del Carmen,* established in 1919 by the *Hermanas Hospitalarias del Sagrado Corazón de Jesús* for poor young girls with bone illnesses, especially tuberculosis and with polio after-effects.[28] The *Sanatorio Marítimo Nacional de la Malvarrosa* was also a hospital for patients with tuberculosis, but as their numbers declined, children with serious polio after-effects were hospitalised there and treated with sun- and sea-bathing. According to Álvaro López Fernández, 'these centres now have a high number of beds occupied by polio patients and, more important, there is no age limit and patients may remain in the clinic until their complete recovery'.[29] The institution was part of a network of four maritime sanatoria, offering primary school education and continuing education for adolescents, sometimes via correspondence courses, along with gendered occupational therapies. The latter, available also to adults, 'entertained them and provided some income to help their economic position, and furthermore had a role that was even more important and more charitable, which was to make them aware of who they were and that they might have a useful part to play in society'. As López put it:

> 'Our mission must not stop when the patient is released from hospital. We must fight to ensure that when he leaves the sanatorium, he can feel like a normal man, capable of filling a post which his character deserves and ready to undertake a full involvement in life.'[30]

Thus natural physical therapies such as heliotherapy were widely used for the inmates of these coastal sanatoria, modelled on predecessors in other European countries. Such therapies were first among medical technologies used in the rehabilitation of polio patients, though surgical procedures were seen by doctors as the only way to achieve a body figure as close as possible to that of a 'normal' child and in certain leg paralysis cases the consensus was for combined use of

---

27 The famous Spanish painter Joaquin Sorolla portrays in 'Triste herencia' a Brother of San Juan de Dios bathing children from the hospital at Malvarrosa beach.

28 www.hospitalariasmadrid.org:8080/hospitalarias/opencms/hospitalarias_valencia [consulted 11.01.2009]; Corbín Ferrer, J.L. La Valencia marinera: del Grao a la Malvarrosa, Valencia, Federico Doménech, 1994, 180-181.

29 López Fernández, A. *Estado actual del tratamiento de la poliomielitis*, Cuenca, Colegio Oficial de Médicos, 1964, 4. Álvaro López Fernández joined the centre in 1932 later becoming its director until his death in 1974. A highly gifted surgeon, he became Regional Head of the Fight against Invalidism in 1936 and Chief of the Physical Medicine and Rehabilitation Service of the Levante Region in 1949.

30 López, 'Estado actual'.

'the knife and the sun'.[31] However other measures were adopted, for example those associated with Kenny from 1940 onwards. She was the most popular and controversial physical therapist of the time who advocated early movement of the affected limbs against the complete rest and immobilisation prescribed by doctors.[32] Her ideas were harshly criticised by the medical profession as a whole but many supported her methods for their common sense and efficacy.[33]

The modernisation of the health system during the Second Republic involved the creation of the Health Statistics Service in 1930 by Marcelino Pascua and the systemised obligatory notification of diseases, which gave rise to further studies on the epidemiology of poliomyelitis, for example during the epidemic in Santander that year. Publications on infantile paralysis acknowledged the good results obtained from serum therapy; the need for compulsory notification; for isolation and disinfection, and for rehabilitation.[34] Shortages of resources limited the impact of therapeutic recommendations by Spanish doctors, but these approximated to ideas promulgated by the permanent Committee of the International Office of Public Hygiene, following the epidemics of 1929 and 1930 in the Netherlands. They included 'the organisation of recourses for neurological clinics, the distribution of convalescent serum, hospitalisation as soon as possible at the State's expense, and the offer of facilities for hydrotherapy and electrotherapy treatment from the end of the acute stage'.[35]

The period between 1929 and 1936 marks the beginning of the 'discovery' of polio victims as a new group of disabled people and the establishment of orthopaedics as a speciality in Spain, raising a new question: what place did a child affected by polio occupy in society? As in other countries, concern for the health and welfare of children increased and the need to protect the physical, mental and moral well-being of those considered at risk encouraged the

31 Nelson, M. Clark. 'Sun or the Knife. Treating children with skeletal and other forms of tuberculosis at Apelviken ca. 1900-1930'. Unpublished paper .

32 Sanz Ibáñez, J.; Sanchis Olmos, V. 'Estudio crítico de los tratamientos de la parálisis infantil'. *Acta Pediátrica Española, 42*, (1945), 587-610; Martín Lagos, F. 'Prevención de deformidades y rehabilitación', in Bosch Marín, J. (dir.). *Aportación española al V Simposio Europeo de Poliomielitis*, Madrid, Dirección General de Sanidad, 1958, 103-104.

33 In Spain the use of hot packs was questioned by González Mas R. 'Rehabilitación del poliomielítico', in González Mas, R. (ed.) *Tratado de rehabilitación médica*, Barcelona, Editorial Científico-Médica, tomo I, 1965, 239. Cohn, V. *Sister Kenny. The Woman who Challenged the Doctors*, Minneapolis, University of Minnesota Press, 1975. See also Oshinsky, D. *Polio. An American Story. The Crusade that mobilized the Nation against the 20th Century's most feared disease*, New York, Oxford University Press, 2005, 73-78.

34 Fernán Pérez, J. *Epidemiología de la Parálisis infantil*, Madrid, 1932, 52-54.

35 Fernández Ruiz-Sánchez, L. 'Comité permanente del Office Internacional de Higiene Pública'. *Boletín Técnico de la Dirección General de Sanidad*, 1930, 777; Fernández Ruiz-Sánchez, L. 'Comité permanente de la Oficina Internacional de Higiene Pública', *Boletín Técnico de la Dirección General de Sanidad*, 1931, 26.

development of numerous institutions and professionals.[36] Schools became the prime arena for the socialisation of children, gradually transforming, in Viviana Zelizer's words, the wage-earning 'non-child' of the labouring poor into the category of the economically worthless pupil.[37] Compulsory schooling revealed children who failed to comply with rules and regulations or were unable to fit in with educational norms. They were often labelled 'abnormal'. This varied and unspecific category included children with problems of adaptation and 'unacceptable behaviour', 'mental handicaps' and children with physical impairments (including sufferers of important muscle-skeletal illnesses such as polio); the latter groups at least considered innocent victims.

The 1940s and 1950s outbreaks

Further poliomyelitis outbreaks occurred at the end of the Civil War, in the 1940s and above all, during the 1950s, coinciding with the Franco dictatorship and suppression of earlier Republican reforms. An exceptional surviving feature was the National School of Public Health in Madrid, whose work mostly continued along Republican-style lines. Excluded from the newly-established United Nations, Spain underwent a period of great hardship, hunger and abject poverty, as one of the poorest and most underdeveloped countries in Europe. For example, compulsory health insurance, introduced in 1942 was not developed substantially until the late 1950s.[38] However, the work of epidemiologists during the

---

36 See Rodríguez-Ocaña, E. (ed.) 'Child Health, a paradigmatic issue in modern history', *Dynamis, 23* (2003), 17-166; Cooter, R. (ed.) *In the name of the child: health and welfare, 1880-1940*, London, Routledge, 1992; Fildes, V. and Marks, H. (eds.) *Women and children first: International maternal and infant welfare, 1870-1945*, London, Routledge, 1992; Appel, R. *Reaching out of mothers: public health and child welfare*, Sheffield, EAHMH Publications, 2002; Gijswitj, M.; Marland, H. *Cultures of child health in Britain and the Netherlands in the Twentieth Century*, Amsterdam, Rodopi, 2003. For Spain: Ballester, R. and Balaguer, E. 'La infancia como valor y como problema en las luchas sanitarias de principios de siglo en España', *Dynamis 15*, (1995), 177-192; Rodríguez-Ocaña, E. 'La construcción de la salud infantil. Ciencia, medicina y educación en la transición sanitaria en España', *Historia Contemporánea, 18* (1999), 19-52; Perdiguero, E. (ed.) *Salvad al niño. Estudios sobre la protección a la infancia en la Europa Mediterránea a comienzos del siglo XX*, Valencia, PUV, Seminari d´Estudis sobre la Ciència, 2004.

37 Zelizer, V. *Pricing the Priceless Child: the changing social value of children*, New York, Basic Books, 1985, 3-21; 208-228. Hendrick, H. 'Constructions and reconstructions of British childhood: an interpretative survey, c. 1800 to the present', in James, A. and Prout, A. (eds.) *Constructing and reconstructing childhood*, Basinsgtoke, Falmer Press, 1990, 35-59.

38 'La Salud pública en la España de la primera mitad del siglo XX', in Atenza, J. and Martínez, J. (eds.) *El Centro Secundario de Higiene rural de Talavera de la Reina y la sanidad española de su tiempo*, Toledo, Junta Central Castilla la Mancha, 2001, 37-38; Rodríguez Ocaña, E. 'The politics of Public Health in the State-Managed Scheme of

1940s prepared a new approach to poliomyelitis, with a re-evaluation of environmental factors and their possible practical implications. In 1946, J. Durich highlighted the tendency 'of clinical cases to occur outside urban centres' and 'at early ages', based on the Mallorca (1932) and Valencia (1942) outbreaks.[39] He noted the importance of environmental features and referred to recent Danish studies on the development of poliomyelitis, where a growing incidence of cases among adolescents and adults was related to the 'general improvement in health and water supplies', which offered fewer opportunities for infection.

The connection between improved hygiene and the epidemic presence of poliomyelitis now became the norm in Spain, no doubt reflecting modern scientific studies, but also allowing Spain to be shown as a country undergoing modernisation and one which might be accepted among western countries.[40] Its active and significant participation in the international fight against polio offered non-democratic Spain the best possible opportunity of alignment with other European nations. In other fields, such as maternal and child health or trachoma, the country might lag behind but in the case of polio, as a result of improved hygiene, sanitation and living conditions, Spain had the consolation of finding itself on an equal footing with other countries.[41] Polio appeared to be an illness of developed countries and, 'as in nearly all the countries with a high level of health care, polio cases tended to rise in Spain while infant mortality fell'.[42]

Healthcare in Spain (1940-1990)', in Löwy, I.; Krige, J. (eds.) *Images of Disease. Science, Public Policy and Health in Post-war Europe*, Luxembourg, European Communities Pub., 2001, 187-210.

39 Durich, J. 'Contribución al estudio de la poliomielitis', *Revista de Sanidad e Higiene Pública*, 20 (7) (1946), 663-700.

40 However, there was no experimental evidence before the late 1950s. Ballester, R. and Porras, M. I. 'El significado histórico de las encuestas de seroprevalencia como tecnología de laboratorio aplicada a las campañas de inmunización. El caso de la poliomielitis en España', *Asclepio*, 61 (1) (2009), 55-80; Báguena, M. J. 'Estudios epidemiológicos y virológicos sobre la poliomielitis en Valencia (1959-1969)', *Asclepio*, 61 (1) (2009), 39-54.

41 Bernabeu, J.; Perdiguero, E. 'At the service of Spain and Spanish Children, Mother and Child: Healthcare in Spain during the first two decades of Franco's Regime (1939-1963)', in Löwy; Krige 'Images of Disease', 167-186; Bernabeu, J. et al. 'Niveles de vida y salud en la España del primer franquismo: las desigualdades en la mortalidad infantil', *Revista de Demografía Histórica, 24* (2006), 181-201.

42 Bosch, J. and Bravo, E. 'Aportación de España a la lucha contra la poliomielitis', in *Aportación española al V Simposium europeo sobre poliomielitis (1958), Madrid, 28-30 de septiembre 1958*, Madrid, Publicaciones 'Al servicio del niño español', Ministerio de la Gobernación, 1958, 45-51.

During outbreaks in 1950, 1952, 1958 and 1959 some 2,132 cases of paralytic poliomyelitis were officially reported.[43] Some research suggested a shift of cases to higher age groups; its prevalence in rural zones or diverging distribution by age groups between urban and rural areas, explained this in terms of population density, levels of hygiene or carriers. However, other studies found no difference in disease incidence in urban or rural environments and continuing predominance in children less than two years, as in the outbreaks in Seville and Santander in 1950 and in Andalusia and most of Spain in 1952.[44] This reopened the question whether poliomyelitis should be considered as a disease of civilisation.[45] It appeared from the 1954 Barcelona outbreak that urban inhabitants were vulnerable, particularly children aged one to three years, unlike the pattern indicated by other researchers.[46] Heavy internal migration from the countryside towards Catalonia, the Basque Country, Valencia and Madrid, with the expan-

---

43 González Rodríguez, P. *Epidemia de poliomielitis en España en 1950*, Madrid, Publicaciones 'Al servicio del niño español', Ministerio de la Gobernación, 1951; Clavero, G.; Pérez Gallardo, F. 'Epidemiología de la poliomielitis', *Acta Pediátrica Española, 8* (2) (1951), 1169-1194; González Rodríguez, P.; Bosch Marín, J. 'La parálisis infantil en España (Estudio del brote epidémico de 1952)', *Revista de Sanidad e Higiene Pública*, 27 (11-12) (1953), 613-622; Pérez Gallardo, F. 'Epidemiología de la poliomielitis en España. Encuesta serológica para la determinación de los anticuerpos antipoliomielíticos en la población española', *Revista de Sanidad e Higiene Pública*, 36 (1962), 501-518; Pérez Gallardo, F. 'Epidemiología de la poliomielitis en España. Aislamiento de los virus poliomielíticos y otros enterovirus', *Revista de Sanidad e Higiene Pública*, 36 (1962), 605-635; Pérez Gallardo, F.; Nájera Morrondo, J. A.; Ruiz Falcó, F.; Nájera Morrondo, E. 'Estudio de los casos y defunciones por poliomielitis, notificados mediante la ficha epidemiológica, en el quinquenio 1955-1959', *Revista de Sanidad e Higiene Pública*, 36 (1962), 374-414; Pérez Gallardo, F.; Nájera Morrondo, J. A.; Ruiz Falcó, F.; Nájera Morrondo, E. 'Epidemiología de la Poliomielitis en España. Estudio de la morbilidad y mortalidad durante los años 1931-1935 y 1940-1962', *Revista de Sanidad e Higiene Pública*, 37 (1963), 454-470; Navarro, 'Análisis de la Sanidad', 179. See also previous figures concerning Madrid, Barcelona and Valencia included in the first pages of this work.

44 Morales, J.L. 'Poliomielitis. Estudio epidemiológico. Profilaxis y tratamiento', *Acta Pediátrica Española, 8*, (1950), 1141-1159. The author, Head of the Provincial Services of Infant and Maternal Health, studied 69 cases of poliomyelitis in Seville (27 in the capital and 42 in the province); Mezquita López, M. [Provincial Head of Health of Almería] 'Consideraciones sobre la poliomielitis y la epidemia de Andalucía durante el año 1952', *Revista de Sanidad e Higiene Pública, 26* (11-12) (1952), 621-640; González Rodríguez, P.; Bosch Marín, J. 'La parálisis infantil en España (Estudio del brote epidémico de 1952)', *Revista de Sanidad e Higiene Pública, 27* (11-12) (1953), 613-622, 618.

45 González; Bosch. 'La parálisis infantil en España', 621.

46 Sales-Vázquez, R. 'Poliomielitis: Epidemiología y profilaxis. A propósito del brote epidémico de 1954 en Barcelona', *Archivos de Pediatría, 5* (28) (1955), 359-397.

sion of slums, once more alerted the medical world to the importance of environmental factors in poliomyelitis epidemics.

During the 1940s and 1950s published work outlined the main characteristics of polio treatment, showing its complexity.[47] Together with serums, physical procedures, Kenny treatment, radiotherapy, electrotherapy, diathermy, spinal galvanic stimulation, some Spanish authors began to stress the advisability of the hospitalisation of patients, from disease control, specialisation and cost considerations. For example the neurologist Izquierdo Rubin, taking the case of the USA as an example, argued for the establishment of specialist centres and hospitals, with a national organisation responsible for therapeutic initiatives.[48] Subsequently, the Decree of 4th August 1947 planned 'Four centres for the fight against poliomyelitis', in Madrid, Barcelona, Seville and Santander.[49] These came under the *Dirección General de Sanidad* (General Board of Health Department), corresponding to the strategy outlined by Izquierdo Rubin, though little materialised until 1951, when an 'Anti-poliomyelitis Service' was founded under the auspices of the General Health Department in Madrid's *Niño Jesús Hospital.*[50] Its outpatient service comprised nurses, instructors or paediatric nurses, and two hospital doctors, the hospital service consisting of a special ward, an orthopaedic surgeon, an intern, a specialist in viruses from the National School of Health, and nurses. However, the ward was not completed until the late 1950s, as polio morbidity reached its peak in Spain.

At this crucial point the National Poliomyelitis Service was also established, following European standards and located in Ward Three of the *Hospital del Rey* (Madrid) and responsible to the General Health Department.[51] Spain's economic penury delayed its official inauguration until 1960, and similarly plans to extend the anti-polio services to deal with provincial outbreaks.[52] Along with *Dirección General de Sanidad* services some provinces had arrangements within the

47 An example of this is Lorente Sanz, A. 'Problemas de actualidad sobre la poliomielitis anterior aguda', in *Libro de Actas de las Jornadas Médicas españolas celebradas en Zaragoza los días 26 al 30 de septiembre de 1943*, Zaragoza, 1944, 935-938.

48 Izquierdo Rubin, J. 'Estudio epidemiológico, clínico y terapéutico de la parálisis infantil. Tercera parte. Tratamiento', *Yatros, 11* (1947), 4-11; 12, 1-10; 13, 1-9.

49 BOE, 14-8-1947, 226, 4564-4565.

50 Porras and Ballester, 'The incorporation of medical technology'; BOE, 25. 4. 1951, 115, 1879.

51 Building work for this Service was only completed in 1959. Dirección General de Sanidad. *Memoria de la Dirección General de Sanidad correspondiente a los años 1957-1958*, Madrid, 1959, 183; ibid. 1959, 9, 81. According to Torres Gost, Director of the Hospital, this decision was taken in the mid-1950s and he travelled to England, Paris (*Hôpital des Enfants Malades*, Granches), Munich (Poliomyelitis Section of the Paediatric Service), Bologna and Scandinavia before designing the National Poliomyelitis Service. Torres Gost, J. *Medio siglo en el Hospital del Rey*, Madrid, Biblioteca Nueva, 1975, 133-134.

52 Some newspapers covered this event. For example, *ABC*, 8 March 1960, 5, 37-38.

Compulsory Sickness Insurance scheme. It appears, for example, that there were special wards within the paediatric section of public hospitals in Valencia, though documentary evidence is needed to confirm oral testimony here.[53] Spanish doctors were well informed of the latest therapies used against polio in more advanced countries, but the country lacked resources and specialists before the 1960s, when they were confined mainly to urban areas.

As yet there was no means of fighting the clinical illness once developed and treatment was still mainly palliative, directed towards the prevention and observation of complications, using natural physical means, physical electrical treatments and iron lungs. [54] By the 1940s the possibility existed of fighting respiratory complications using the Drinker Respirator, a tank type respirator and later known as an iron lung, or respirators in the form of a sleeveless jacket or cuirass. Noting American experience, Izquierdo Rubin reported on the potential treatment of respiratory polio, though 'in the majority of Spanish hospitals we do not as yet have access to these magnificent devices'.[55] However, some apparatus was installed in the specialised services and centres and the 130-bed National Poliomyelitis Service at the *Hospital del Rey* offered 'two artificial respiration rooms, one with seven iron lungs and the other with three positive and negative pressure respirators for use via tracheotomy', complemented by 'a set of cuirass ventilators for respiratory rehabilitation and assistance to patients recovering from respiratory paralysis'.[56] The Poliomyelitis Service of the Child Jesús Hospital in Madrid, the Malvarrosa National Maritime Sanatorium in Valencia and other anti-polio centres also had similar equipment, according to papers presented at the Fifth European Symposium on Poliomyelitis held in Madrid in 1958.[57]

In 1950 the Valencia City Council had brought in 'the first iron lung imported in Spain'.[58] This was installed in the *Casa de Socorro of Ruzafa* and, according to the paediatrician Dámaso Rodrigo, was the only device of this kind in

53 These technical resources were possibly located at the University Clinic (first in the Provincial Hospital, and after 1960 at the Clinic Hospital), the Provincial Hospital or at the General Sanjurjo Hospital (opened in 1956).

54 Trueta, J.; Wilson, A. B. K; Agerholm, M. *Poliomielitis. Principios y prácticas de su tratamiento*, Barcelona, Ed. Juventud, 1957, trad. castellana del inglés, 65 (the authors have used a Spanish translation of the English original).

55 Izquierdo, 'Estudio epidemiológico', 2.

56 This Service had foreign and national iron lungs. Dirección General de Sanidad. *Memoria de la Dirección General de Sanidad correspondiente a 1959*. Madrid, 1959, 9, 81.

57 López Fernández, 'Estado actual', 6; Bosch and Bravo, 'Aportación', 48.

58 Concerning No-Do, see: Tranche, R. and Sánchez-Biosca, V. No-Do. *El tiempo y la memoria*. Madrid, Cátedra/ Filmoteca Española, 2002; Medina Doménech, R.M.; Menéndez Navarro, A.'Cinematic representations of medical technologies in the Spanish official newsreel, 1943-1970', *Public Understanding of Science, 14* (2005), 393-408.

Valencia.[59] Iron lungs were used most commonly on polio patients unable to breathe and wholly dependent on the equipment and nursing staff.[60] They were all imported and their installation was presented as yet another technological advance by the Francoist government, notably at the 1958 Symposium. The occasion had been carefully prepared by the regime as a health and publicity showcase. Papers by Spanish representatives illustrated five fronts in the Spanish campaign against poliomyelitis: research; vaccination campaigns; education and propaganda; treatment for those affected with a network of iron lungs in provincial capitals and some towns, with rehabilitation services.[61] Much was yet to be implemented, however, and most therapeutic resources were located in towns.

Polio vaccination campaign in the sixties

During the 1960s the Franco regime encouraged economic growth, hoping that prosperity would provide social peace and compensate for the lack of democracy. Rapid economic and population growth was accompanied by new *Seguridad Social* (Social Security Insurance) legislation in December 1963,[62] seeking to unify the different systems of prevention and public protection and widen

---

59 Rodrigo, D. 'Pasado, presente y futuro de la parálisis infantil (Compendio histórico). Lección inaugural del curso 1954-55'. *Anales de la Universidad de Valencia, 28*, Cuaderno 1, (1954-55), 164.

60 First widely used in the 1930s, this was a rigid cylinder into which the patient was placed, with positive and negative pressure applied at regular intervals. The iron lung has attracted debate in the literature on medical technology, as an example of 'half-way technology' [Maxwell, J. 'The iron lung: halfway technology or necessary step'. *New England Journal of Medicine, 285* (1971), 1366-1388], offering a technical fix for a disease that could not be cured. Such technologies tended to be expensive, in contrast with truly effective 'definitive technologies' based upon the inner working of the disease (in the case of polio the Salk and Sabin vaccinations). Stanton, J.: 'Suported lives'. In Cooter, R.; Pickstone, J. (eds.) *Companion to Medicine in the Twentieth Century*, London, Routledge, 2003, 607-609. For Patients' experiences see: Gould, T. *A summer plague. Polio and its survivors*. New Haven/London Yale UP, 1995, 309-310; Sass, E. Polio´s Legacy. *An oral history*, Lanham, University Press of America, 1996.

61 Bosch and Bravo, 'Aportación', 45-51.

62 Its implementation was delayed until 1967. García Padilla, M. 'Historia de la acción social: Seguridad Social y asistencia (1939-1975)', in *Historia de la Acción social pública en España. Beneficencia y Previsión*, Madrid, Centro de Publicaciones Ministerio de Trabajo y Seguridad Social, 1990, 397-447. Benjumea Pino, P. 'Sanidad y desempleo', in *Historia de la Acción social pública en España. Beneficencia y Previsión*, Madrid, Centro de Publicaciones Ministerio de Trabajo y Seguridad Social, 1990, 449-472; Rodríguez Ocaña, E. 'La asistencia médica colectiva en España hasta 1936', in *Historia de la Acción social pública en España. Beneficencia y Previsión*, Madrid, Centro de Publicaciones Ministerio de Trabajo y Seguridad Social, 1990, 321-359. Rodríguez, 'The Politics of Public Health', 195-198.

State social support.[63] By now serological surveys and epidemiological studies enabled the authorities to assess the magnitude of the polio problem and its distribution by age-group, urban or rural environment and socio-economic level.[64] There were slight differences in urban and rural areas, with 'those between one and two years' particularly affected in urban and intermediate areas, although in the northern coastal region 'medians were slightly higher than two years old'.[65] With some 80 per cent of polio patients being children under five years of age, the need to extend vaccination to all children, whether in towns, suburbs or country areas was clear.

The first mass immunisation campaign with oral polio vaccine was carried out by the General Department of Health in 1963. Two rival vaccines had been developed in post-war America, Jonas Salk´s Inactivated Polio Vaccine (IPV) and Albert Sabin´s oral vaccine (OPV). Interestingly, Salk´s vaccine was tried in the USA whilst Sabin´s vaccine was trialled in the Soviet Union as the Cold War Powers looked to prophylactic vaccines as defensive weapons. Preparations for the Spanish campaign were made from late 1961 with further efforts to prompt favourable public reception and ensure implementation of the plan by 1963.[66] Accordingly:

> 'The national campaign was carried out in two phases, the first between 20th November and 20th December 1963 and the second in April 1964. [...] A little before each of the phases a propaganda campaign was carried out in which all the proper means collaborated (press, radio, television, etc.) [...] The organisation of the campaign was planned with great thoroughness in order to ensure it reached the most remote corners of the country, through the introduction of mobile units made up of a doctor and three nursing assistants who carried the vaccine from the provincial health departments to all urban, suburban and rural areas.'[67]

---

63 The later Franco regime has been seen as *Estado autoritario paternalista (Authoritarian Paternalistic State)*, which others prefer to call *Estado autoritario de Bienestar*. See Muñoz de Bustillo, R. (comp.) *Crisis y futuro del Estado de Bienestar*, Madrid, Alianza Editorial, 1989, 184-189. Comín, F. 'Las formas históricas del Estado de Bienestar: El caso español', in *Dilemas del Estado de Bienestar*, Madrid, Fundación Argentaria, 1996, 42. This social advance was the basis of the Welfare State established after the restoration of democracy.

64 Pérez Gallardo, 'Epidemiología de la poliomielitis en España. Encuesta serológica', 501-518.

65 Pérez Gallardo *et al.* 'Estudio de los casos y defunciones por poliomielitis', 396.

66 See, for example, *ABC*, 14. 5. 1960, 62; 5. 6. 1960, 101; 21. 12. 1960, 89; 2. 4. 1961, 73; 22. 7. 1961.

67 Mezquita López, M. *Evaluación de los resultados de la primera campaña de vacunación contra la poliomielitis por vía oral en España*, Madrid, Dirección General de Sanidad, 1965, 21.

Sabin was invited to Spain, giving a conference in Madrid in February 1963, followed by Pierre Lépine, the head of the virology service of the Institute Pasteur of Paris.[68] Press coverage of these visits aimed to win public support for mass immunization with OPV, as in other countries.[69] Within Spain, the government sought to flag up these signs of modernity and demonstrate the nation's equal footing with other countries in the worldwide fight against polio, with the NODO, the Spanish newsreel, even including the Soviet Bloc in its reports.[70]

The results of the mass campaign were excellent.[71] Whereas the 1955-1963 average of reported cases was 1,733 per annum, there were only 155 in 1964. Yet subsequent research pointed to infancy as the highest period of risk, suggesting that underlying problems were poverty and lack of access to vaccination.[72] The relationship of polio with rural migration to the cities was also established and once again environmental factors were suggested in the development of outbreaks. It was therefore proposed that the Epidemiological Survey System should coordinate the laboratory studies of the *Centro Nacional de Microbiología, Virología e Inmunología Sanitarias of Majadahonda* (Madrid) with socio-economic ones. This approach emerged as Spain entered a new historic phase: the *transición democrática* (democratic transition), which implied signi-ficant changes.

In the atmosphere of concern and hope of the early 1960s a pioneer example of relevant associationism from civil society emerged with the launch at the *Club Internacional de Prensa* (International Press Club) in Madrid of the *Asociación Española de la Lucha contra la Poliomielitis* (Spanish Society against Polio) on 19 June 1963. Chaired by the Duke of Alba, this comprised people of high social standing with a management board including Professor Ciriaco Laguna. It described itself as a kind of charity, seeking to complement and support the work of the state with 'medical advice in order to ensure the total vaccination of Spanish children and the provision of all the affection, and human kindness that society can offer in the recovery process'.[73] The charity

---

68 Sabin, A. *Erradicación de la Poliomielitis: estado actual y perspectivas futuras. Conferencia dada en Madrid en el Consejo Superior de Investigaciones Científicas*, Madrid, CSIC, 1963.

69 *ABC*, 5.2. 1963, 50; *ABC*, 7.2. 1963, 53-54; 10.2. 1963, 59; 16.3. 1963, 69; *Las Provincias*, 19.2. 1963, 11.

70 Ballester, 'La presentación internacional'. The archives of NO-DO (acronym of 'Noticiario y Documentales Cinematográficos') reveal how news on polio vaccination events was shown. See also, Ballester, R. 'Imágenes de la vulnerabilidad: Las Fuentes fílmicas de la poliomielitis en España'. In Ortiz Gómez, T. et al. (coords.) *La experiencia de enfermar en perspectiva histórica*, Granada, Universidad de Granada, 2008, 335-339.

71 Mezquita, 'Evaluación', 37-38.

72 Nájera Morrondo, 'Análisis epidemiológico'.

73 *ABC*, 21.6. 1963, 48.

provided medical care but also kept vigil over spiritual, cultural, moral, economic and social interests and its mainly urban organisational model was similar to that of the Spanish Society for the Fight against Cancer.

Supported by *Cáritas Nacional* (a section of Caritas Internationalis) and with state collaboration, the Spanish Society against Polio established four schools in Madrid (two for boys and two for girls) for child victims of polio in March 1964.[74] Almost ten years later it established its own facilities (*Centro de Educación Especial para Niños Deficientes Motóricos)* behind the *Hospital del Niño Jesús* in Madrid, with premises provided by the *Organización Nacional de Ciegos Españoles* (ONCE) which were more suitable for children affected by polio.[75]

Conclusions

In studying poliomyelitis in rural and urban Spain, three stages may be observed. Between 1890 and 1930, in the context of socio-political crisis and with Spanish society fully aware of the need for in-depth sanitary reforms, the illness acquired greater visibility as isolated outbreaks occurred, early publications appeared, innovative epidemiological surveys were carried out and polio was included among legally notifiable diseases. Infections were analysed and strategies of intervention were developed following the usual hygiene issues: deplorable sanitary conditions, the role of vectors, and the predominance of unhealthy rural and poor urban areas. Serum therapy, hospitalisation and rehabilitation became key therapeutic elements – especially in urban areas – and the period marked the 'discovery' of polio victims as a new group of disabled people.

The epidemic phase of the illness in the 1940s and 1950s saw considerable increases in polio morbidity, a partial shift towards towns and the political use of epidemiological data. Coincidentally, the Franco regime's eagerness to change its external image and to seek international influence meant that polio became considered as 'a disease of civilisation'. This period marked the creation of a network of preventive and therapeutic public health services devoted to polio sufferers. Finally, the first mass immunisation campaign occurred in the 1960s, using OPV and based on scientific data provided by serological surveys and the

74 The Society had a School Council which included the general director of Primary Education and representatives from the Ministries of National Education, Work and the Interior. *ABC*, 24.3. 1964, p. 49-50. However, its chairman was the Duke of Alba and the general secretary was Mª Dolores Gascón de Ramos, both of the Spanish Association against Polio. The School Council was responsible for the appointment of teachers with the required qualities to look after children with polio, but also the payment of their compensation for housing.

75 *ABC*, 14.2. 1973, 119.

epidemiological studies carried out by the General Department of Health. These data confirmed the need to extend vaccination to all children up to five years of age in all areas. We also find in Madrid the first example of relevant associationism, in civil society. But the relative failure of later vaccination campaigns, compared to other western countries, led to renewed attention to underlying features such as poverty and the poor sanitary conditions of disadvantaged social groups such as migrants from the countryside to the cities.

FOOD SAFETY, THE RURAL/URBAN DICHOTOMY AND VALENCIAN SOCIETY 1850-1930

Ximo Guillem-Llobat

The second half of the nineteenth century marked a period of intense changes in the food chain. The process of industrialisation and urbanisation experienced by many areas of the European continent was crucial for the reorganisation of each of the stages included in the production, distribution and commercialisation of foodstuffs. These changes occurred at a different pace in each European state but finally they all went through this same process. Thus food production became mechanised; foodstuffs started to be sold in an increasingly processed form; new products were invented and disseminated among consumers; distribution networks experienced rapid expansion; and there was a revolution in retailing.[1]

Each of these changes in the food chain contributed in one way or another to the consolidation of a new context for food safety. In this chapter I will first analyse generally and using a case study, how these major changes influenced the development of food quality and safety, comparing urban, semi-urban and rural areas. I will consider the rural/urban divide through the double divide described in the Conference of European Statisticians held in 1964.[2] On that oc-casion the participants in the conference agreed that those areas with more than 10,000 inhabitants would be deemed 'urban', those with less than 2,000 re-garded as 'rural', with the interim grouped as 'semi-urban'. As we shall see in our particular case study, the Valencian Country, changes in the food chain were experienced first within urban areas, only to be introduced much later in rural areas, with some middle-size municipalities having an interim position.[3]

This is not to say that such a model can be applied everywhere or that the urban/rural dichotomy involved only one set of relationships concerning food safety problems. However, focusing upon the relationship between industrialisation of the food chain and new food safety problems in the Valencian Country,

---

1 Guillem-Llobat, X. *El control de la qualitat dels aliments. El cas valencià en el context internacional (1878-1936)*, Valencia, PUV (CD-ROM), 2008

2 Champion, T.; Graeme, H. *New Forms of Urbanization. Beyond the Urban-Rural Dichotomy,* Aldershot, Ashgate, 2004.

3 The Valencian Country is also known by names such as Valencian Community or Valencian Kingdom. Indeed, the name of the region has been constantly discussed in recent decades. For more information see: http://en.wikipedia.org/wiki/Names_of_the_Valencian_Community.

the link between urbanisation, industrialisation and new food safety problems is demonstrable.

A second part of the chapter considers the measures introduced to tackle new food safety problems. In this sense, Valencian urban, semi-urban and rural areas also featured different major strategies. Thus, the comparative frame will allow us to evaluate and question the magnitude of the benefits resulting from the imposition of the new methods of control, increasingly based on chemistry and on the search for standards in the composition of foodstuffs, as the basis for further discussion.

The establishment of a new food chain in the Valencian Country

The Valencian Country experienced the aforementioned transformation of the food chain some time later than in more industrialised countries.[4] Changes would, nevertheless, take place at all stages of the food chain including production, distribution and retailing.

Around 1900 not many food industries were operative and, indeed, it was mainly from 1914 that food production and processing were transformed.[5] However, the transformation of the food chain had its origin in initiatives that can be traced back to the 1830s. For instance, Martínez Gallego has highlighted the enormous influence of the abolition of regulations that reserved the possession of mills to the large landowners of the old regime.[6] Since the abolition of these regulations in 1834 many new mills were created for the production of flour, oil, rice, etc., followed, in the second half of the century, by an intensive growth of milling associated with the use of new technology and energy sources. Moreover, these changes then prompted the establishment of new industrial sectors such as those linked to the production of soup pasta.

The development of an ice industry in the second half of the nineteenth century was also very important for the establishment of new food industries producing soft drinks, beer, ice creams and conserves. Refrigeration techniques later made possible the development of the meat industry, though this occurred in the twentieth century.

The medical topography of Benetússer, then a small village of less than 2,000 inhabitants near Valencia, illustrates the importance of the developing meat in-

---

4 Soler, V. 'L'economia valenciana al tombant de segle', *L'Espill* 2 (1999), 124-144.

5 Santacreu Soler, J.M. *L'economia valenciana durant la guerra civil: protagonisme industrial i estancament agrari*, Valencia, Alfons el Magnànim, 1992.

6 Martínez Gallego, F.A. *Desarrollo y crecimiento. La industrialización valenciana 1834-1914*, Valencia, Generalitat Valenciana, 1995.

dustry.[7] In the 1920s two meat factories, the *Frigorific La Plata* and *La Catalana Industrial*, operated in the village. The former was established by Santiago Aguar, a pioneer in the refrigeration of processed pork products in the region, and involved in the first Valencian factory of this type before he established his own business in Benetússer.[8] In his new factory, he succeeded in appropriating the technology used to freeze meat; a methodology that was quite difficult to control and a previous restriction on this industry.[9]

The production of chocolate and confectionery, and of alcoholic beverages, also underwent a process of mechanisation with the appearance of new factories. The industrialisation of their production was enhanced in Valencia during the 1920s with the development of a new culture of leisure time. A period of economic prosperity favoured the establishment of new specialised shops, cafeterias and bars as a popular alternative to *casinos* (clubs) and *ateneus* (arts and sciences associations).[10] This promoted consumption in the capital city as well as in some semi-urban areas such as Ontinyent and Xàtiva.[11]

The new food industries appeared mainly in urban centres such as Valencia and Alicante but in semi-urban areas and small villages located near important urban centres, food industries were also established. For instance, municipalities of around 10,000 to 15,000 inhabitants such as Vila-real also experienced the establishment of new food industries such as factories for soft drinks, sugar refining and for orange exporting. Villages of 2,000 inhabitants or even less, like Benetússer, might produce chilled meat, spirits, coffee, vegetable oils, soft drinks, along with fruit and vegetable exports, although remote areas had still not experienced this transformation in food processing activities. Thus Ròtova, a

7 Navarro Soler, V. *Topografía médica de Benetúser. Obra laureada por la Fundación Röel, en el concurso celebrado por el Instituto Médico Valenciano*, Valencia, Imprenta José Olmos, 1927.

8 Medical topographies were written by local physicians and even though they were the product of a detailed study usually evaluated by an expert commission (in the case of the topography of Benetússer, the text was successfully evaluated by the jury of the Röel Prize of the *Institut Mèdic Valencià*) they could include certain vague remarks. In this sense, Vicente Navarro's testimony may not be enough to be sure that there were no other factories in the Valencian region similar to the one where Aguar worked. However, we can feel confident to state that, in any case, he would be introduced in this profession in the context of the origins of this kind of meat industry in the Valencian region.

9 I use the concept of appropriation as an alternative to reception in order to emphasize the active role of Aguar in the introduction of the freezing techniques.

10 Girona, A. 'Una nueva forma de vivir: la urbe como modelo de atracción', in *La ciudad moderna. Arquitectura racionalista en Valencia*, Valencia, 1998.

11 Martínez Gallego, F.A. *Desarrollo y crecimiento. La industrialización valenciana 1834-1914*, Valencia, Generalitat Valenciana, 1995.

traditional rural village with a very low level of industrial activity even around 1920 had only limited works linked to the export of agricultural produce.[12]

In general terms, the process of industrialisation of food production experienced in these areas eventually had important consequences as regards food safety problems. Mainly in urban centres, food safety problems increased as the links of the population with agriculture, ranching or other activities of the primary sector diminished.[13] The distancing of urban populations from food production activities made them less familiar with the origin of foodstuffs and less capable of identifying pure foods. Country people in contrast could still identify frauds by the organoleptic features of foodstuffs and were less exposed to the general increase in food adulteration experienced in most of the European states during the second half of the nineteenth century.[14]

There were also important changes in the distribution of foodstuffs. Rail networks and the installation of chilled chambers in trains and ships from the late nineteenth century progressively increased the distances involved in food marketing. In Valencia, the arrival of fresh (or not so fresh) fish from Barcelona became subject to regulation by the Civil Governor after continual complaints from people about its poor quality.[15] However, foreign foodstuffs did not flood the Valencian market in the way they did in, say, British cities. Around Valencia, importations of foodstuffs were even less, as was stated in 1920. Several mayors of Valencian municipalities and some presidents of farmers unions and

---

12 Izquierdo Sánchez, J. *Topografía médica de Rótova y pueblos anejos a su distrito,* Imp. Francisco Vives Mora, 1911.

13 The decrease in the urban food production activities accelerated as competition with rural and foreign producers increased. Features such as urban pollution, the price of urban land and the passing of new regulations restricting the presence of animals in the city also contributed to the reduction of these activities in urban areas such as those of Great Britain (for more information see: Atkins, P.J. 'Is it urban? The relationship between food production and urban space in Britain, 1800-1950' in *The Landscapes of Food. The Food Relationship of Town and Country in Modern Times*, Helsinki, 2003). In Valencia the link of the population to the primary sector was progressively reduced, especially during the 1920s and 1930s with further decline in the number of agricultural workers and a progressive increase of its industrial labourers (for more information see: Girona, A. 'Una nueva forma de vivir: la urbe como modelo de atracción'. In: La ciudad moderna. Arquitectura racionalista en Valencia. Valencia, 1998). Nevertheless, the city of Valencia still conserved quite an agrarian character if we compare it to other European cities. Indeed in 1930 there was still around a 40% of the population dedicated to the primary sector.

14 Atkins, P.; Lummel, P.; Oddy D.J. (eds.) *Food and the City in Europe since 1800*, Aldershot, Ashgate Publishing, 2007.

15 Arxiu Municipal de València. 'El Sr. Governador Civil manifiesta habérsele denunciado que en los trenes correo y mixto de Barcelona llegan a la estación del Norte remesas de pescado en malas condiciones'. Secció 1a, subsecció D, classe II, subclasse K, caixa 14, núm. 55, 1911.

associations met to complain that rural areas were usually excluded from the distribution network of rice, flour and oil; these products were mainly sent to the capital city and smaller municipalities depended only on their own production.[16]

The extension of the food chain over longer distances entailed new problems in certifying food safety as food suppliers became more anonymous and consumers less able to secure reliable suppliers. Again though, possibilities of food fraud differed between rural and urban areas. People in the countryside directly controlled more stages in food production, leaving a narrow margin for adulterators to act. Fewer foodstuffs were imported and even these were usually sold in less-processed forms as more people still had direct access to food production. There were fewer food shops and rural areas tended to be excluded from distribution networks, with correspondingly fewer rural consumers.

The final stages of the food chain also saw important changes with a late nineteenth and early twentieth-century retailing revolution affecting most European cities.[17] New regulated markets and fixed food shops began to replace older forms of hawking, which also became more regulated or was banned.[18] This new organisation of retailing had interesting consequences for food safety issues. New food shops might promote the consumption of foodstuffs imported from other regions and abroad, affecting food quality where they were subjected to greater risk of adulteration.[19] Yet fixed shops were better regulated and entailed the building of new trust relationships between customer and proprietor: the shopkeeper could not be anonymous and needed to secure customers' confidence and loyalty.[20] Yet, this new trust in shopkeepers could have a positive or negative consequence on the quality of foodstuffs, depending on the balances

---

16 Arxiu de la Diputació de València. [Meeting of mayors and presidents of agrarian unions and associations of the Valencian Province to deal with the distribution of rice, oil and flour] E.11, caixa 53, 1920.

17 See Spiekermann, U. 'Rationalisation as a permanent task. The German food retail trade in the twentieth century', in *Food Technology, Science and Marketing: European Diet in the Twentieth Century*, East Linton, 1995; Oddy, D.J. 'From corner shop to supermarket: the revolution in food retailing in Britain, 1932-1992', in *Food Technology, Science and Marketing: European Diet in the Twentieth Century*, East Linton, 1995.

18 In the city of Valencia regulations of the food market can be traced back to the early modern period, when the mustassaf was the institution in charge of food inspection. Since the imposition of the Castilian laws in the 18th century the mustassaf was substituted by the more limited figure of the Almotacen, but food control still continued. However, in the 19th century major changes were introduced in food legislation in order to adapt regulation to the new situation to which the change in the food chain had lead.

19 As stated when dealing with the changes in food distribution, the importation of foodstuffs from longer distances entailed new problems in food safety as food suppliers became more anonymous and consumers less able to secure reliable suppliers.

20 Ferrières, M. *Histoire des peurs alimentaires: du Moyen Âge à l'aube du XXe siècle*, Paris, Editions du Seuil, 2002.

struck in retailer-customer relations. It could be positive because shopkeepers might be reluctant to cheat the customers they wanted to secure but, on the other hand, as customers became more confident they lost former abilities to identify fraud by their own means.

Once more such changes had greater impact in the city than in the countryside. From the second half of the nineteenth century reforms were introduced in the markets of Alicante and Valencia, aiming to improve hygiene conditions attendant upon the commercialisation of food.[21] In semi-urban areas such as Gandia and Vila-real a similar transformation of retailing was also underway (the respective municipal archives still keep interesting documents which certify the existence of controversies related to the hygienic and commercial regulation of the markets).[22] Specific information for semi-urban areas such as Dénia suggests that by 1900 many new and bigger grocers were established in the centre of the town but not yet in surrounding or rural areas.[23] Small villages nearby had neither modern markets nor grocers' shops and there was a more usual consumption of self-produced foodstuffs.

The importance of autoconsumption in the Valencian rural areas was highlighted by contemporaneous authors. Medical topographies of several Valencian villages stated that local populations were never in danger of starving as they always had access to self-produced foodstuffs.[24] Such autoconsumption has

21 The new markets of Alicante would be created in 1842 and 1884, but by the end of the century some reports still criticized their hygienic conditions. For more information see Bernabeu-Mestre, J.; Perdiguero Gil, E. 'Salud, alimentación y consumo', in *Canelobre: revista del Instituto de Estudios Juan Gil-Albert* 43 (2001), 104-117. The market of Valencia, on the other hand, was already praise by J.B. Peset i Vidal in his medical topography of Valencia and its conditions would still be improved by the beginning of the 20th century with arquitectonic reforms introduced and the construction of a new building.

22 In the case of Gandia see, for instance: Arxiu Municipal de Gandia (AMG). [Demand of a change of location of the market to a ventilated area outside the walls of the city]. carpeta: 'mercat 1847-1936', 1854; AMG. [Merchants of the municipal market write a letter addressed to the Mayor and denouncing that peddlers are working inside the market with no license]. carpeta: 'mercat 1847-1936', 1925; AMG. 'Expediente instruido para la regulación de la venta ambulante en la población, en cumplimiento de la O. del Ministerio de la Gobernación de 25 de Mayo y Decretos de 11 de Julio de 1934'. carpeta: 'mercat 1847-1936', 1934. In the case of Vila-real see, for instance: Arxiu Municipal de Vila-real. [Report on the hygienic conditions of the slaughterhouse and the municipal market and a proposal of reforms addressed to the Municipal Health Board]. 86 (1)/1923, 1923.

23 Calvo, J. *Agricultura, industria y comercio en la Dénia del siglo XIX*, Alicante, Universidad de Alicante, 2003.

24 For instance, the medical topographies of Meliana (see: Durán Martínez, J. *Topografía Médica de Meliana*, Valencia, Imprenta de la Revista Valenciana de Ciencias Médicas, 1915), Sollana (see: Vera Verdú, F. *Topografía médica de Sollana*, Valencia, 1926) and Ròtova (see: Izquierdo Sánchez, J. *Topografía médica de Rótova y pueblos anejos a su distrito*, Imp. Francisco Vives Mora, 1911) stated that the population had direct access to a

always been difficult to measure, particularly using a socio-economic approach to food history and, therefore, its impact may well have been understated.[25] Nevertheless, we know it was a usual practice and probably resulted in lower overall levels of food adulteration in rural areas, given that self-producers were unlikely to adopt such practices.

Foods adulterated and consumed

In the reorganisation of the food chain another interesting change came with the invention and introduction in the market of new industrial foodstuffs such as margarine, saccharin, sauces, corn flakes, and prepared foods. These required special quality controls, since their novelty and levels of processing offered greater opportunities for fraud than the traditional fresh foods. Grocers in large and medium towns were selling most of these foodstuffs by the 1920s but in rural Valencia there were few shops and the consumption of these products was less. This fact contributed, once more, to the establishment of important differences in the magnitude of fraud in rural and urban areas.

Nevertheless, these new foods were not among the most adulterated in the Valencian Country. Reports detailing the activity of the municipal laboratories and the medical topographies throw some light on the main foods adulterated in that region. There was a difference in the intensity of adulterations and in the types of foodstuffs more adulterated between areas. In urban areas, adulterations were mostly detected in bread, flour, chocolate, milk, wine and sweet drinks and foodstuffs. In rural areas these foods were less adulterated. Bread, for instance, was frequently analysed at the municipal laboratory of Valencia during the 1920s and 1930s. By then most bread consumed in towns was baked outside the home and its production might involve use of low quality flour or excessive proportions of water. In rural areas such as Ròtova bread was more frequently

great amount of varied vegetables and fruits, which were grown by them. Moreover, the author of the medical topography of Meliana insisted on the importance that those frogs and snails directly caught in the fields near the town had on the population's diet. In the medical topography of Sollana the author also referred to the hunting of country rats and to some fishing for autoconsumption. We can also consider the domestic breeding of poultry and small mammals for autoconsumption. The importance of this source of food was highlighted, for instance, by the author of the medical topography of Ròtova. Finally, we can refer to the medical topography of Tavernes de la Valldigna, which stated that local peasants would produce almost all their food and they would only buy oil, chickpeas and some secondary commodities.

25 In this sense, Florent Quellier has criticized important studies on food rations such as those of the school of Annales for not having considered the importance of autoconsumption in the population's diet (Quellier, F. 'Le jardin fruitier-potager, lieu d'élection de la sécurité alimentaire à l'époque moderne', *Revue d'Histoire Moderne et Contemporaine*, 51 (2004), 66-78).

homemade, according to the local medical topography and, therefore, not so usually adulterated as in the city.[26]

In the medical topographies of Valencian rural villages the most usual products suspected of being adulterated were condiments, with spices, sugar or salt specifically mentioned in Ròtova, Alberic and Meliana respectively. These were no more adulterated than their urban equivalents but they represented some of the few foodstuffs that most rural inhabitants bought in shops. Their imported condition would determine their greater probability of being adulterated, as suggested above. Contemporaneous authors observed this: for example, the medical topography of Alberic stated that local olive oil, sold in private houses, was not usually adulterated but that imported oil, bought at the shop, might well be.[27]

Urban and rural differentials in food fraud were noted by physicians and chemists in their participation in international congresses and publications. Thus one of the main Valencian forerunners of modern food quality control, Vicent Peset Cervera, said in 1881: 'Today everything is being falsified, everything is being adulterated, ... more so in the big centres of population, where the commercial transit is so big'.[28] Nevertheless while food adulteration was then becoming more noticeable, it was still less extensive than in more industrialised north-European countries.[29]

The organisation of a response to food fraud

By the beginning of the twentieth century food safety was already an important medical and commercial issue in the Valencian Country. Greater food adulteration was highlighted by renowned authors such as the pharmacist and pioneer of modern food analysis in Alicante, José Soler i Sànchez. In 1897 he noted its spread to the south of the Pyrenees and predicted its growth to levels that existed to the north.[30] However actions to improve food control were already underway, notably in regard to markets and slaughter-houses.

---

26 Izquierdo Sánchez, J. *Topografía médica de Rótova y pueblos anejos a su distrito*, Valencia, Imp. Francisco Vives Mora, 1911.

27 *Topografía médica de Alberique* (ca. 1922).

28 Peset Cervera, V. *Proyecto de un Laboratorio de Higiene Pública de Salubridad Municipal*, Valencia, Imp. de Juan Guix, 1881.

29 The distinction between the impact of fraud in rural and urban areas can also be appreciated in the interventions of the Spanish and Swiss delegates, Dr. Fernandez-Caro and Dr. Ferrière respectively, in the debates on food safety that took place at the international congress of hygiene and demography held in Vienna in 1887 (see: *VI Congrès International d'Hygiène et de Démographie a Vienne (du 26 septembre au 2 octobre 1887)*, Vienne, 1887.

30 Soler Sanchez, J. *Análisis y ensayos de los alimentos, de las bebidas y de los condimentos*, Alicante, Establecimiento Tipográfico de Vicente Botella, 1897.

During the first half of the twentieth century, many Valencian towns experienced the renovation of old markets or the building of new ones, and hygiene conditions surrounding food sales were subjected to further regulation, using new municipal licenses and through the hiring of special market inspectors such as those of the *Junta Municipal d'Avituallaments* (Municipal Food Board). Similarly, further controls were introduced regarding perishables such as fish, meat or milk.[31] The construction of slaughterhouses was strongly promoted as early as 1849 by the Valencian Civil Governor after he visited many of the towns and villages. However, as noted by Josep Lluís Barona and Joan Lloret, very few municipalities immediately responded to this demand, so reform took decades to be achieved.[32] The need for hygienic buildings to contain the market or the slaughterhouse was no less in rural than urban areas. Generally, however, the application of reform regulations might reflect the greater resources of larger municipalities. Smaller villages with smaller budgets had probably greater difficulties in carrying out improvements, at the cost of difficulties in preserving food safety.

In the latter decades of the nineteenth century a major change in the regulation of food safety came with the establishment of chemical and bacteriological analysis. Previous detection of food fraud had depended on the study of the organoleptic features of foodstuffs. Merchants and food producers were closely associated with particular foodstuffs and could identify better than anyone, using their expertise and the different senses, whether a particular sample could be considered of good quality.[33] However, chemical analysis became more important, especially after increasing amounts of chemical compounds were used to adulterate foodstuffs in more subtle ways. Yet methods for fraud detection were not solely guided by the supposed superiority of the technical or chemical approaches since other factors were also important. These included the professionalisation of chemistry; the consolidation of increasingly influencial chemical societies; new experimental and instrumental trends in biomedical disciplines; and the advantage of chemical analysis in the debate due to its greater terminological and conceptual complexity (the advantage of asymmetry).[34]

31 For instance, in Gandia fish was regulated through some particular rules passed in 1914. Meanwhile, milk production would also undergo special inspections in Vila-real after the passing of the municipal hygiene rules of 1908.

32 Barona, J.L. and Lloret Pastor, J. 'La higiene dels aliments i els escorxadors. Dos aspectes de la higiene pública a la societat valenciana en els període entre segles', in *Polítiques de salut en l'àmbit municipal valencià (1850-1936)*, València, PUV, Seminari d'Estudis sore la Ciencia, 1999.

33 Stanziani, A. *Histoire de la qualité alimentaire: XIXe-XXe siècle*, Paris, Editions du Seuil, 2005

34 Guillem-Llobat, X. *El control de la qualitat dels aliments. El cas valencià en el context internacional (1878-1936)*, Valencia, PUV (CD-ROM), 2008.

In Europe, the substitution of the methodology had its main turning point in the establishment of municipal laboratories during the 1870s and 1880s. These became the main authority in determining whether a food sample had to be considered adulterated. Moreover, the passing of new food regulations made the use of chemical analysis in food control even more necessary as it promoted the standardisation of foodstuffs in a way that only chemical analysts could reveal whether a particular foodstuff fulfilled the required standards. In the city of Valencia the municipal chemical laboratory was established in 1881, followed by a municipal laboratory in Alicante in 1887.[35] Such laboratories were limited to towns of a certain size, however. The General Health Instruction of 1904 stipulated the need to create a municipal laboratory involved in food analysis in towns with populations exceeding 25,000 inhabitants, reduced to 10,000 inhabitants by a revised order in 1908. Smaller towns and villages were left to rely on individual professionals, such as the municipal veterinary, pharmacist or physician who, if incapable of certifying the quality of a sample, were required to send it to the city laboratory. Thus, apparently, in both urban and rural areas the new emphasis upon chemical analysis carried out in municipal laboratories was dominant.

However, the smaller municipalities, those in rural areas, might have had more difficulties in the application of the new methodology due to their inferior local services or practitioners and to their dependence on outside services, those of the city. Moreover, the 1908 order was not properly applied: some urban and most semi-urban areas were not able to change completely to new forms of fraud detection. Only Valencia and Alicante had active laboratories for the analysis of foodstuffs and the latter resource was modest. The other Valencian provincial capital, Castelló, had more than 25,000 inhabitants in 1900 but lacked these facilities and, for instance, in 1908 several samples of soft-drinks were sent to the laboratory of Valencia by the Civil Governor of Castelló.[36] The 1908 Order required the establishment of a municipal laboratory in towns of more than 10,000 inhabitants but it was not properly applied and towns such as Xàtiva, Vila-real and Gandia still lacked their own facilities. In the case of Xàtiva the mayor received a letter from the Board of Health in November 1911

35 Guillem-Llobat, X. 'El paper dels laboratoris municipals valencians en el control de qualitat dels aliments (1881-1936)', in *Actes D'Història de la Ciència i de la Tècnica* 1 (2008), 293-300.

36 Arxiu Municipal de València. 'El Sr. Gobernador civil de la provincia remite para su análisis en este Laboratorio Municipal seis botellas de gaseosas remitidas por el de Castellón, procedentes de Nules y Castellón'. Sèrie Vària, secció 1a, subsecció D, classe IV, subclasse D (1908(2a)). núm 34 and 37, 1908.

that stated the obligation of the municipality to create a municipal laboratory in accordance with previous food rules, although this had no immediate outcome.[37]

Consequently there was heavy dependence on the city by rural and semi-urban areas in relation to food control. In Vila-real, now with more than 15,000 inhabitants, the local authorities instead of creating a laboratory passed municipal hygiene regulations that established this dependence in 1908. These assigned to the municipal pharmacist food analysis tasks, but stated that cases posing difficulty were to be sent to the provincial laboratory.[38] As in Vila-real, many other villages established similar dependence relationships with the city and these were noticeable when considering the origin of the samples analysed in the laboratories of Valencia and Alicante. The municipal laboratory of Valencia received samples from Alzira, Gandia, Castelló, Nul·les and Godella, while the municipal laboratory of Alicante analysed samples sent from Novelda, Elda, Vila Joiosa, Elx, Dénia, etc.

Municipal veterinarians, pharmacists and physicians also got involved in these analysis tasks. Where there was no active municipal laboratory the pharmacist was usually the main authority in the analysis of food samples, as is clear from the municipal ordinances of towns such as Vila-real. Similarly we know of the analyses carried out by the municipal pharmacist of Sagunt, Eduard Balbó,[39] and his equivalent in Xàtiva, José Ramón Sanchis.[40] Veterinarians would normally be involved in the inspection of animals and the analysis of meat but, occasionally, they also examined other foodstuffs in the market and might be in charge of the analysis of commodities such as milk. In Xàtiva, the pharmacist José Ramón Sanchis reported that he had not analysed milk samples because that was a task assigned to veterinarians.[41] Municipal physicians were less involved in food analysis, although one in each town was named as Municipal Hygiene Inspector, the top official of the municipal hygiene board and in charge of food quality control, though the analysis would normally be done by the pharmacist of the municipal hygiene board. It is significant that the programme

---

37 Arxiu Municipal de Xàtiva. [Letter of the Valencian Board of Health and addressed to the mayor of Xàtiva. It pointed out the need to establish a municipal laboratory in the town] V.1.2.3. Sanitat – Expedients i correspondencia, 1911.

38 The latter reference to a provincial laboratory that would analyse the samples coming from rural Valencia has already been stated in other municipal ordinances. However, in the end it seems that the municipal laboratories of Valencia and Alicante were in fact the ones that analysed the aforementioned samples. The provincial hygiene institutes would be established later on, already in the second and third decades of the twentieth century, and they were not especially involved in food analysis.

39 Barona and Lloret Pastor,'La higiene dels aliments'.

40 Arxiu Municipal de Xàtiva. 'Inspección farmacéutica Municipal Játiva 1941' V.1.2.3. Sanitat – Expedients i correspondencia, 1941.

41 Arxiu Municipal de Xàtiva. 'Inspección farmacéutica'.

required to pass competitive examinations for the position of municipal health inspector in 1930 did not feature food analysis to any major extent.[42]

In rural areas municipal pharmacists, veterinarians and physicians to some degree contributed to the control of food quality through the new methodology of fraud detection. However, they remained dependent on the city laboratories when the sample to be analysed showed some special complexity. As Casadevante and Sanfeliu stated in their 1933 book *Técnicas de Laboratorio. Análisis de Alimentos. Análisis Clínicos*,[43] these rural professionals could not afford expensive treatises on food analyses and lacked the technical means needed to carry out the analysis proposed. However Casadevante and Sanfeliu's book filled a gap in their training as it was affordable and described methods of analysis that could be carried out with the materials available to them.

With the intention of filling the gap in pharmacists' training other initiatives were also promoted in Valencia. Special courses held in the Provincial Hygiene Institute in 1931 consisted of 50 lessons, 15 of them specifically dedicated to the analysis of foodstuffs. This improved the training of rural pharmacists who previously had to prepare largely unaided for competitive examinations. Such measures also aided the chemical approach to food control in rural areas but here the municipal pharmacists or physicians had many other duties. Moreover, as Casadevante and Sanfeliu stated, their methodology might differ from that applied in the city laboratory, being more dependent upon organoleptic studies of foodstuffs and on the use of simple instruments such as the microscope.[44]

This dependence of municipal pharmacists on organoleptic methods meant that in urban and semi-urban areas lacking a municipal laboratory the techniques for food quality control would differ from those of the city. In smaller villages this would be still more obvious as they even had difficulties in securing the presence of a municipal pharmacist. Indeed, the General Health Instruction of 1904 considered that villages of less than 2,000 inhabitants would have to share the municipal pharmacist with other neighbouring villages. Therefore, limitations in the application of the chemical approach to food control would be even greater in those rural areas.

---

42 Palanca, J.A. 'Programa de los ejercicios oral y escrito para oposiciones a plazas de Medicos titulares Inspectores municipales de Sanidad' *Boletín del Instituto de Higiene de la Provincia de Valencia* (1930), 10.

43 Casadevante and Sanfeliu. *Técnicas de laboratorio: Análisis de alimentos. Análisis clínicos*, Madrid, Antonio Marzo, 1933.

44 Casadevante and Sanfeliu, 'Técnicas de laboratorio'.

Conclusions

The rural-urban dichotomy has been challenged by present and past authors on numerous occasions.[45] However, in this study, the double divide as established at the 1964 Conference of European Statisticians seems useful. It fits quite well to the three contexts of food safety regulation outlined, when modified to describe villages of 2,000 people or less, those with 10,000 to 15,000 inhabitants and cities of more than 50,000 inhabitants. The categories reflect three different realities in relation to the dimensions of food safety problems and the services provided to tackle them.

However, the proximity to important urban centres was also a key feature as a determinant of food quality control. Thus a combination of two factors, the number of inhabitants (population) and proximity to the city (location), seems crucial in determining the particular scenario of food regulation in a particular area. The influence of population size and proximity to a major city was intimately related to the different levels of industrialisation of societies. The latter transformed not only food production but also its distribution and commercialisation. In turn, these changes influenced food safety in various ways, but generally, where the change in the food chain was most marked, so were the problems associated with food fraud.

In that context the size of the municipality also largely determined the establishment of different models of food control. While the cities were the forerunners in the introduction of the new chemical approach to food quality controls, rural areas had to reinvent traditional organoleptic methods. This configuration will allow us to study in further researches the relative contribution of chemical analysis to food safety. Similarly, when considering food safety in later periods, it will feature prominently in efforts to evaluate the contributions of marginal rural science to mainstream science.

---

45 A historical testimony of the rural controversy can be found in Cavaillès, H. 'Comment définir l'habitat rural?', *Annales de géographie*, 45 (1936), 561-569. Moreover, an introduction to the current controversy in Pratt, A.C. 'Discourses of Rurality: Loose Talk or Social Struggle?' *Journal of Rural Studies* 12 (1996), 69-78.

TOWN AND COUNTRY: THE STAKES OF INFANT AND CHILD HEALTH POLICY IN FRANCE 1860-1940

Catherine Rollet[1]

Studies of infant mortality generally show high nineteenth-century urban rates, reflecting poor living conditions and inflows of migrants from the countryside. Analysing this feature at the beginning of the 1930s, K. Stouman, former statistician of the League of Nations Health Committee, referred to the 'urban mixer' which, 'crushing the primitive rock of ancient local traditions creates the new mortar which will make the future'.[2] This amalgam of different populations resulted in 'a real disaster as regards infant mortality'.[3] Thus Swedish infant mortality progressively declined but in Stockholm it remained high, sometimes exceeding 300 per 1,000 births. Economic development and political stability did not improve the situation in the capital before the late nineteenth century when it fell to seven per cent below the Swedish national average.[4] Similar trends were discernible in Berlin but not in Paris: due to the wet-nursing system, Bertillon, the Director of the Parisian statistics bureau, had given up any idea of publishing mortality rates.[5] Stouman's 'urban mixer' had paradoxical effects, initially causing higher infant mortality in towns but then working to reduce it. The evidence was clear for countries like Sweden and Germany, but not so for France.

This study focuses on the image that contemporaries had of the countryside. It argues that, during the period between the Second Empire and the World War Two, there was a turnaround in attitudes towards rural areas. Initially these involved assumptions concerning the cultural backwardness of the countryside, belief in technical progress and concerns over the exploitation of the countryside by the towns via the system of wet nursing. While efforts were directed toward improving the situation in urban communities with hospitals, clinics, etc., rural mothers and children were merely under supervision without access to health care or social services. The 1874 Roussel Law focused only on wet-nursed babies in the countryside, not on the countryside as such.[6]

---

1 The author wishes to express her thanks to Julie Rollet for carefully re-reading her English translation.

2 Stouman, K. 'Le redoutable seuil de la vie. Description du cadre démographique de la mortalité infantile', *Bulletin trimestriel de l'organisation d'hygiène*, SDN, Vol. III, 4, December 1934, 615.

3 Stouman, 'Le redoutable', 616.

4 Stouman, 'Le redoutable', 618.

5 Stouman, 'Le redoutable', 619.

6 Rollet, C. *La politique à l'égard de la petite enfance sous la Troisième République*, Paris, PUF/Ined, 1990, 131-136.

However, by the early 1920s rural areas, which had paid a high price in the war, were rehabilitated; the advantages of fresh air, water and sun were recognised and their special needs, involving issues of isolated villages, long distances, poor and large families, were taken into account in new measures. Table 1 provides the schema adopted in this chapter and demonstrates the most important shifts during the period under consideration.

Table 1. General frame of analysis

Characteristic of Period	1874-1890	1890-1914	From 1914
Approach	Medical and social supervision, individual lessons; repression of abuse	Milk supply; mass education; prevention of diseases; use of modern technology (radiology, sterilisation, vaccinations)	To supervise, to educate, to cure
Type	Doctors' visits to wet nurses	Infant health centres; milk depots	Visits and infant health centres
Means	Medical and administrative inspection	Prevention and cure in urban infant health centres and hospitals; philanthropy (charities)	Integration of public and private initiatives, to associate medical and social supervision
Professions	Medical inspectors; social work inspectors	General practicians and physicians in hospitals	Health visitors, physicians, social workers
Categories of children	Children separated from their parents (fostered in rural areas and abandoned children)	Middle and working class children	All children: A health book for every child (1939)
Area of intervention	Rural areas	Towns	Urban and rural areas

A critical approach to rural health: the problem of infant mortality

France remained a predominantly rural country in this period, the 'end of the countryside' occurring only after World War Two.[7] Specific features such as dispersed population and difficulty of access to villages or hamlets in the mountains, help to explain rural deficiencies in schooling and health infrastructure, not least as physicians, teachers and other professions involved in child welfare, education or health, preferred town comforts and the financial resources of the bourgeoisie to underpin their activities.

7 Weber, E. *La fin des terroirs. La modernisation de la France rurale 1870-1914*, Paris, Fayard, 1983.

The golden age of the rural areas from a demographic point of view was during the 1820s and 1830s, before mid nineteenth-century urbanisation and industrialisation led to the decline of living conditions and population in the countryside. The urban bourgeoisie exerted its domination over the new working classes and the peasantry but its approach to rural populations was both contradictory and ambiguous. On the one hand the countryside represented nature, fresh air, physical exercise, a healthy life, down-to-earth common sense and country ethics. Jean-Jacques Rousseau had conceptualised the countryside as a naturally invigorating resource to fight off the toxic miasmas of the town, a place for rest and health improvement, an ideal location for childbirth and childrearing, far from urban noise and stress. This option was indeed chosen by some bourgeois families, as seen below.[8] More important, though, was that abandoned babies were given to families in the countryside to be fostered, and in Burgundy and Brittany wet nurses were recruited for the needs of the urban bourgeoisie.[9] Yet the rural world was also considered as boring, backward, prejudiced, unhygienic, illiterate, and poverty-stricken. The mid nineteenth-century image that townspeople created of the countryside and rural populations, bourgeoisie of peasants, and educated people of illiterate ones, is well illustrated by the debate from 1865 concerning infant mortality, child health and possible improvements.

In *Lessons on infant hygiene* Dr. Jean-Baptiste Fonssagrives demonstrated this ambiguity towards the rural, asking: 'which is the best environment for infant vitality, town or countryside? Nine out of ten would without hesitation answer: the countryside'.[10] This was formerly his opinion, but now he thought neither the city nor the countryside, but the small town which had the advantages of both.

In the ensuing debate rural-based physicians discussed the subject of fostered children and what they called the 'nursling industry' and, like many civil servants, focused on the factors associated with high infant mortality. The attached map of infant mortality in the period 1857-1866 was presented to Members of Parliament by Adolphe Bertillon in 1874, and it made a strong impression.[11] A large area north of the Loire, the departments near the Rhône valley and the regions of Savoie and Provence appeared as shockingly unhealthy. However, a key feature was that all deaths of fostered babies were recorded in the

8 Rollet, C. *Les enfants au XIXe siècle*, Paris, Hachette, 2001, 80-81.

9 Monot, C. *De l'industrie des nourrices et de la mortalité des petits enfants*, Paris, 1867; Brochard, *De la mortalité des nourrissons en France, spécialement dans l'arrondissement de Nogent-le-Rotrou (Eure-et-Loir)*, Paris, Baillière, 1866.

10 Fonssagrives, J.-B. *Leçons d'hygiène infantile*, Paris, Delaye, 1882, 34-36. Based on lectures given in Montpellier, where he was Professor of Medicine,

11 Rollet, C. *La politique à l'égard de la petite enfance sous la Troisième République*, Paris, PUF/Ined, 1990, 38-42.

department where they occurred, rather than the department of birth, thereby raising rural mortality.

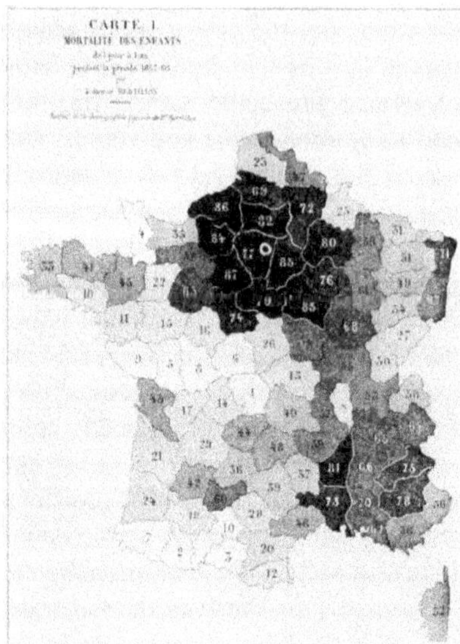

Bertillon demonstrated that infant mortality 1855-66 in ten departments where babies were fostered was 20 per cent for local babies but 52 per cent for fostered Parisian babies. This turned political attention towards the living conditions of rural fostering families: their bad and crowded housing; lack of fresh water; earthen floors; lack of lighting and heating and unhygienic cohabitation of people and animals, were all denounced. Similarly with the incidence of child accidents and threats from animals, fire, falls, changes in temperature etc and, finally, the lack of basic education on hygiene and the persistent influence of all kinds of prejudice and superstition (see *L'Illustration* below).

Any real attack upon excessive infant mortality in towns or countryside called for fundamental economic and social change. Instead, the bourgeois solution focused upon the mortality of fostered children as the attackable problem. And even though some of the excessive mortality among fostered infants reflected bad conditions surrounding pregnant mothers and childbirths, the dominant preference was to concentrate upon rural, poor fostering families. For example, rural prejudice was problematised. In 1875 a Nevers' physician summarised the prejudices surrounding infant-related diseases in Central France.[12] He described popular beliefs relating to birth, breastfeeding, infections and convulsions, also denouncing popular prejudices around vaccination, which was considered dangerous and useless.[13] Similarly, local correspondents of Academy of

12 Subert, *Préjugés du Centre de la France relatifs aux maladies des enfants*. Nevers, 1875. The newspaper *La jeune mère. Education du premier âge*, of Dr Brochard, is also a mine of information about the so called prejudices of the countryside: see the chapters concerning mol paws, scabs on the head, infant diseases, etc.

13 Among these was that May was seen as the best month for vaccination, that the large 'boutons' (spots) were the best to prevent smallpox, that vaccine on the arm of a child was dangerous etc. Later, under the Third Republic, many authors, through the distribution of small booklets, tried to eradicate popular prejudices and to educate mothers and wet nurses on the basics of scientific knowledge. See for example articles published in the *Almanach illustré à l'usage des jeunes mères*: Dr Emile Bessières, 'Les affections intestinales.

Medicine criticised arrangements for fostering, notably breastfeeding habits, clothing, and cradles.[14] Such analyses counterposed two types of population and knowledge, rather like contemporary observations by anthropologists on attitudes and beliefs of immigrant populations living in a completely different environment.[15]

Only a few observers urged a more thoroughgoing study of high infant mortality. They noted the transformations affecting the rural world, particularly the loss of rural industry ('proto industry'), incomes and livelihoods, and the exploitation of rural families by urban and richer ones. They highlighted the refusal of rich mothers to breastfeed their infants and the impossibility for working mothers to do this when day care centres were rare; with minimal allowances for single mothers, the lack of equipment and poor education in rural areas. Yet a discourse acknowledging the respective situations of town and countryside was not pursued: what remained was the notion that rural areas were unhealthy and, in particular, that fostering families were dangerous.[16]

The engravings from *Illustration* reflect this general mindset, with seven drawings intended to shock the reader over the fate of innocent infants suffering the poverty, ignorance and prejudices of their foster parents. Each engraving was distinctly violent, emphasising that nurslings were exposed to danger at the wet-nurse's home. Thus one baby was suffocated by a cat, another burnt to death and a third was devoured by a pig. Meanwhile a woman and man (called 'accomplices') were carrying babies like packages; elsewhere a woman plunged a baby into a miraculous source and, finally, a baby lay in a grave. One result of this debate was the organisation of State supervision to guarantee the interests of both urban and rural families and their children.

Préjugés populaires', *Almanach...*, 1881, 21-28; Dr Emile Bessières : 'Des préjugés populaires sur les maladies de l'enfance. Lettre d'un père à sa fille. Des fièvres éruptives', *Almanach...*, 1888, 43-46; Dr Dubousquet-Laborderie, 'Préjugés au sujet de l'allaitement maternel. Ses avantages, et dangers de l'allaitement mercenaire', *Almanach...*, 1892, 36-38; Dr Bessières, d'Egreville, 'Hernies et vers intestinaux. Préjugés populaires', *Almanach...*, 1895, 40-42.

14 'Rapport de la Commission de l'hygiène de l'enfance', *Académie de médecine*, 1873, 1874.

15 Comparing the observations of physicians in the 1870's and those made by anthropologists in the 1990's takes on meaning: we find the same type of observation about clothing, feeding, crying, common infantile diseases, ritual prevention ceremonies etc.). See for example Ruspoli, S., L'acculturation dans les pratiques de maternage: quels enjeux dans la relation familles-institution de la PMI (Protection maternelle et infantile). Rapport ACEPP/MIRE, March 1996.

16 Rollet, *La politique à l'égard*, 107-108.

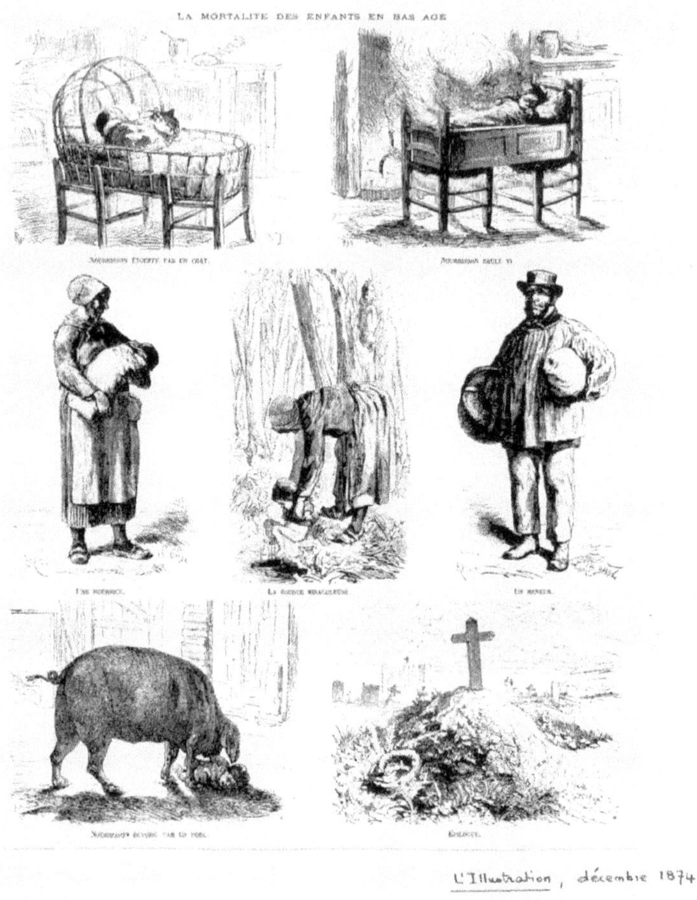

Source: *L'Illustration,* 1874, December 12th

The doctor/inspector: 'an irascible fault-finder' (1874-1890)

Following the Franco-Prussian war, the first infant protection policies were introduced under legislation proposed by Théophile Roussel on 23rd December 1874. Compulsory regular and paid inspections by medical practitioners of wet and dry nurses caring for children aged less than three years were under-taken by volunteer physicians, supported by departments and public welfare inspectors.[17] Yet only rural wet and dry nurses were to be visited while urban families with wet nurses at home went unaffected, barring a revision of legislation dating back to 1762 that a mother could only work as a wet nurse if her own baby was at least seven months old.

How was the supervision organised and perceived and did attitudes change over time? The annually reported observations of physicians and inspectors exist for the whole period until World War Two. However, the foster families' point of view was not recorded in such documents, though examples can be drawn from sources in western France, notably Normandy, Maine and Ile-de-France.

To convince wet nurses of the benefits of the recommended methods, doctors used extracts from 'elementary advice for mothers and wet nurses' issued by the Academy of Medicine in 1872 and as leaflets or posters displayed at town halls.[18] A visiting physician might use such a leaflet to open up a discussion with the nurse, a method probably more efficient in regions such as Normandy where women were more literate than in southern France. More substantial publications such as Brochard's *De l'art d'élever les enfants* (1866) rarely reached the rural public, being considered by the Inspector for the department of Côte-d'Or in 1880 as too long and scholarly. In inexpensive booklets such as *La Jeune Mère,* (1873), and *Almanach illustré de la jeune mère* (1875-1878), Brochard adopted a simpler style with illustrations, though this probably appealed more to the urban middle class.[19]

Education through word of mouth, practical lessons, reading, but above all through treatment was probably more effective. Foster families often experienced their first contact with scientific medicine in this way, compared with use of traditional bonesetters, nuns and home remedies. The free doctor's visits were in the best interests of the wet nurses, their nurslings and their own children and, while doctors focused upon prevention during their visits, initially they also treated sick babies (for which they were reimbursed by the department) and others they encountered, for example the wet nurse's baby or an older child, usually

---

17 De Luca, V. *Aux origines de l'Etat-Providence. Les inspecteurs de l'Assistance publique et l'aide sociale à l'enfance (1820-1930)*, Paris, Ined, 2002.

18 Rollet, *La politique à l'égard*, 344-345. This was updated in 1873, 1885 and 1892.

19 Rollet, *La politique à l'égard*, 346. A doctor/inspector wanting to inform wet nurses from the Paris suburbs published in 1890 the first issue of the *Bulletin for Wet Nurses*. However, the publication was short-lived and never got as far as the departments.

at their own expense. It is likely that this medical care constituted an important step in the process of the medicalisation of rural families for, as one doctor noted, 'the most important consequence of the application of the law is the willingness of wet nurses to call for a doctor at the very outset of disease in a nursling'.[20]

Wet nurses soon saw the advantages of regular visits by doctors who could affirm from eye-witness accounts that babies were not maltreated, but reared along with the other children in the family and, in many cases, doted on. The doctor was closer to the foster family than to the biological family, which rarely visited and often lived far away, and he legitimised the work of the foster family, which was held in higher repute than the biological parents. As one foster mother remarked to a visiting doctor, with a certain air of annoyance, 'the care I provide this baby is a lot more than I'm paid for'.[21] Doctors readily recognised devotion to duty, attachment and warmth even if they thought maternal love was reserved by the wet nurses for their own children. Maternal love for a foster baby, explained one doctor, came only in the case of abandonment by its parents, through their death or neglect, though some admirable, devoted women did not hesitate to keep foster babies despite a large drop in salary. Thus one 'who had cared for a baby for seven months without wages, she decided to bring him back to the parents who were greatly displeased and declared that they did not know what to do with him. They so intimidated the woman that, out of love for her nursling, and fearing that the baby would be ill-treated by his parents, she took him back home with a distinctly lighter purse'.[22]

Of course, nurslings' sufferings did not suddenly disappear, given the persistence of economic misery, ignorance and neglect. One inspector observed in 1886: 'the nurses who are too poor can often get by during the breastfeeding period but when the moment of weaning arrives, it is no longer possible to leave a baby in these homes because of the risk of lack of care and cleanliness and of bad feeding'.[23] A year later he noted the phylloxera crisis affecting vineyards, which 'brought widespread misery, forcing people to search for all possible means of survival'. Ill- treatment by wet nurses and parents still occurred but the image of fostering babies had significantly changed. Nurses and doctors progressively adjusted their methods of operating, which undoubtedly had a positive effect on the survival and wellbeing of infants. Thus 'The physician had

20 Eure-et-Loir, 1883. References to the medical reports (*Enfants assistés et protection des enfants du premier âge*) used are cited with the name of the department and date of the publication.

21 Rollet, C. 'Au temps de la loi Roussel: nourrices et médecins-inspecteurs. Biberon et petit-pot. L'allaitement dit "artificiel" au temps de Pasteur', in *Nourrice ou crèche. Histoire de l'enfant gardé au 19e siècle*, Musée Château Saint-Jean, Nogent-le-Rotrou, 1998, 25.

22 Aisne, 1893.

23 Côte-d'Or, 1886.

been the enemy of the wet nurse. Now, it's the contrary' and even, 'cleanliness, once a luxury for the poor, is becoming apparent in the most humble of homes'.[24]

From new technologies to socio-demographic analysis (1890-1914)

By 1914 the image of the countryside was changing with the Roussel Law, falling infant mortality and the multiplication of scientific studies. Inspectors of public welfare and physicians compared rural and urban mortality, depicting the countryside as abandoned by a largely town-orientated policy, with rural families, once seen as the guilty party, now considered as victims.[25] Towns had indeed benefited from the practical application of Pasteur's principles with baby clinics, milk depots, and maternity services with incubators and specialised physicians, day-care centres and kinder gardens for infants. These were unheard of in the countryside, though some inspectors had tried to utilise portable baby scales, offer safe bottles to foster women, or provide sterilisers for milk. Thus inspector Barthès (Calvados) searched for an area supplier for suitable sterilisers and asked for departmental finance, but sterilisers were difficult to use and so wet nurses quickly abandoned them. In the department of Côte d'Or, each foster mother taking a baby into care from the hospital was given a steriliser and instruction in how to use it.[26]

Similarly, bodies such as the 'Association des Dames Mauloises' in the department of Seine-et-Oise, lent incubators to young mothers with hypotrophic (very low weight) babies.[27] Some established services for pregnant women at home, providing labour equipment and cradles which could later be disinfected and lent out again. Modern follow-up methods for newborn babies were proliferated in this way, though such examples were still rare before 1914 and innovations, even when encouraged by some inspectors, were not always adapted to rural life.

Other initiatives, like that taken by the Mayor of Villiers-le-Duc, doctor Morel, in the department of the Côte d'Or, met opposition from department civil servants. Doctor Morel wanted to generalise the 1893 laws on free medical assistance and the Roussel Law.[28] Since 1883 the township had provided free

---

24 Côte d'Or, 1896, 1900.

25 Renouard, J.-M. *De l'enfant coupable à l'enfant abandonné. Le traitement scial et politique de la déviance* (From the guilty child to the abandoned child. Social and political treatment of deviancy), Païdos, Histoire, Centurion, 1990.

26 Côte d'Or, 1899; De Luca, V. and Rollet, C., 'Nouvelles pratiques de puériculture. Etat des savoirs, acteurs, résistances et avancées. France 1880-1930'; Bourdelais, P. and Faure, O., *Les nouvelles pratiques de santé. XVIII-XXe siècles*, Belin, 2005, 67-88.

27 Pecker, *La puériculture par l'assistance à domicile*, Paris, Baillière, 1900.

28 Archives départementales de la Côte-d'Or, 19 X 3e 5. Many thanks to Virginie Lanaud for these references.

medical and pharmaceutical treatment to the poor; with a first aid post offering basic surgical equipment, bandages and medicine. Families were advised about feeding their children and milk sterilisers and baby scales were provided. Madame Altenbach, Assistant Manager at the midwife school, was sent to Paris to be trained in the use of doctor Tarnier's artificial incubator, working 'with keenness and intelligence'.[29] These arrangements received special authorisation from the prefecture in 1895 and were renewed in 1898 but were rejected by the Prefect in 1901 as incurring expenses not legally required. The Mayor disputed this, obtaining support from the Minister of Welfare, since the measures taken undoubtedly served 'to effectively protect the lives of infants' as none of the babies cared for on the basis of his method had been lost during the previous decade.[30]

If this example illustrates the difficulty of implementing new methods in rural areas using older legislation, we next consider examples of how rural physicians worked; in particular concerning the establishment of infant clinics, as in Finistère in Brittany in 1907. Here the new Inspector of Public Welfare set up ten infant clinics and foster mothers and mothers who received public aid to provide for their infants were obliged to bring their babies to clinics if they lived within three kilometres. The clinics operated in local town halls on Sunday mornings and by 1909, 55 such centres were open and 6, 829 infants seen, 4, 084 of these actually brought freely by their parents. However, doctors' notes confirm uneven results: the clinic in Briec, near Quimper, was an instant success and cases of diarrhoea and eczema had diminished, but Doctor Gaumé found that 'it is very difficult to keep up motivation with these country people when no payment is involved'.[31] Doctor Hébert in Plozevet was more optimistic: the town hall's meeting room was 'well-aired, well-lit, very warm and easy to clean' and babies did not suffer from the transport to the centres, for even during winter storms were rare. Even so, some mothers would have to travel far to reach a health centre and minimum numbers of families in each catchment area were essential. The alternative for rural doctors was to visit families at home. Doctor Hébert supervised breastfeeding as artificial and premature feeding was practised and nearly all babies brought to the infant health centre were fed in this manner. Fortunately the quality of the milk in the area was very good and a milk depot was unnecessary: it was sufficient to recommend boiling the milk for a long time, which was common practice.

---

29 Côte d'Or, 1891.

30 He maintained his interpretation of free medical assistance and the Roussel Law, but had to limit publicity at the town hall. Irritated by the fact that he had been opposed by the Prefecture services, he threatened to refer to the Conseil d'Etat and inform Doctor Adolphe Pinard who was backing him.

31 Finistère, 1907.

To attract families, the physician, at the end of each consultation offered free advice and medicine coupons, which were greatly appreciated. Indeed in 1914, the department assembly agreed that a fee of 0f25 be distributed to each woman presenting a baby at the clinic.[32] Mothers were also keen to weigh their babies: the 460 children presented in 1909 included slightly more boys than girls, reflecting the sex ratio at birth; with more babies in January, March, June and July than from September to December, reflecting seasonal work patterns. From July women were very busy with agricultural work: harvesting and making saltwort with wrack, and it was during this season that cases of summer diarrhoea broke out, causing many deaths.[33]

In 1907 Doctor Hébert felt that, 'in the fight for the survival of human seed, a lot needs to be done, despite the improvements already achieved, in this country full of secular prejudices, of embedded routine, of built-in apathy and rooted scepticism'. A doctor in Quimper observed that a premature infant could have been saved by an incubator, whereas another doctor in Quimperlé felt that some mothers came to the clinic with healthy babies to be weighed, simply to report the results to all their friends.[34]

The Finistère example is not unusual and other rural departments, aided by departmental assemblies and often on the instigation of the Inspectors of Public Welfare, tried to adapt a system of infant clinics to the countryside. The initiative in the department of Yonne was taken by a local physician, Doctor Marois, but the Inspector of Departmental Public Welfare attributed its success to himself. As early as 1904, Doctor Mocquot had set up a clinic in Appoigny with such good results that he then felt obliged to open five others.[35] Subsequently Doctor Marois admitted to the department assembly in April 1904 that he 'could not have foreseen how easy it would be to convince our wet nurses to present the nurslings regularly to a special health centre. I was quite apprehensive about it and I quoted some critics concerning this innovation with the aim to run it down'. Yet 'resistance had disappeared and the habit of presenting babies to the clinics had been adopted by foster women'.[36]

Rural mothers understood the advantages of weighing babies when this also provided the occasion to consult a specialist. In many rural departments this was practised reflecting fears over depopulation and excessive infant mortality. In the Central Mountains, in the department of Pas-de-Calais and in Provence, such

---

32 Finistère, 1913.

33 Finistère, 1909.

34 Finistère, 1907.

35 Budin, P. 'La ville de Paris et la mortalité infantile', *Revue philanthropique*, 1904, t. 14, 412. Budin takes Doctor Marois initiative as an example to extend infant clinics to the whole country; cf. Rollet, *La petite enfance*, 374-384.

36 Yonne, 1911.

clinics had been opened and facilitated the medical inspectors' work. It was recognised, for example, that in transporting baby scales to foster families the scales lost accuracy and the visit took a long time, whereas it was more practical to bring families to a centre, which made the work of the physician easier, according to the wet nurses.[37]

Nevertheless, many difficulties remained in some rural areas, especially in the south of France. Added to the natural obstacles related to climate, transports, and isolated villages, there was often a strong resistance in the minds of the people. The infant clinics failed in departments such as Dordogne, Haute-Savoie, Lot-et-Garonne, Jura and even in Oise, to the north of Paris. A report concerning the Alpes-Maritimes confirmed that local mothers did not want babies to be weighed; they did not accept the public consultation; they refused to undress their babies and ridiculed the doctor while doing this.[38] Southern women saw infancy as an exclusively private matter and opposed any attempts involving medicalisation of families at the hands of male doctors. In addition, weighing babies was considered dangerous and mothers opposed it in the region of Savoie until the 1920s and similarly in regions of western France, such as the Ille-et-Vilaine, Mayenne and Morbihan, where populations were dispersed.

In 1901, A. Balestre and A. Giletta de Saint-Jospeh, from Nice, published a well-known study on urban infant mortality, based on the *Statistique des villes de France et d'Algérie* data.[39] In 681 French towns, there were 292,363 infant deaths over the five years to 1897, of which they alleged three quarters were preventable.[40] No-one had made similar calculations for the countryside, however, and Bertillon's 1874 map was too dated usefully to serve this purpose. However, L. Cruveilhier, a small country town mayor and a physician, attempted to do so using statistics he had himself gathered from ministerial offices, departments and municipalities, showing that rural areas often suffered from higher infant mortality than towns.[41] In particular, he noted how small numbers and the question of fostered children distorted the situation. Comparing infant mortality rates for towns like Nice, Besançon, Nîmes, Saint-Malo, Guéret, Limoges and rural regions around these towns produced ambiguous results because of the migration of babies after their birth. But calculating new rates for the districts of Limoges and Nice by removing the deaths of children born in a town other than their place of death revealed higher mortality for several rural

---

37 Rollet, *La politique à l'égard*, 395.

38 Rapport... Hygiène...enfance, *Bulletin de l'Académie de Médecine*, 1910, 10.

39 Doctor A. Balestre was the director of municipal board of hygiene of Nice.

40 Balestre, A. and Gilletta de Saint-Joseph, A., *Etude de la mortalité de la première enfance dans la population urbaine de la France de 1892 à 1897*, Paris, Doin, 1901.

41 Cruveilhier, L. 'La mortalité infantile à la campagne', *Revue philanthropique*, 15 novembre 1911, 7-41.

villages around Limoges (16 out of 82 villages an excess of 15 per cent or more) and similarly for the Nice region (16 out of 74 villages, an excess of 23 per cent and above). Thus, the addition of fostering inflated rural infant mortality rates and decreased urban ones, though rural infant mortality was sometimes intrinsically higher than in urban areas. He concluded that 'rural mortality is often as high as in urban areas and sometimes higher than in industrial towns'. Since most of the diseases causing death were preventable, especially in the countryside, he called for a real 'sanitary crusade' in the municipalities, villages and towns, as advocated by the Senator Paul Strauss.[42]

The changes in analysis are also related to the new vision of the rural situation as the first results of child and maternal welfare efforts in towns were observed, as detailed in Figure 2 and Table 2 below, although separate data for rural and urban areas are not available.

The great 1911 crisis, with hot summer weather causing intestinal diseases, was obvious and focused attention on towns and countryside alike.[43] It affected the whole of northern France and an area south of the Massif Central, resulting in more than 29, 000 victims among children less than three years old.

Figure 2. Trends in mortality rates at 0, 1 and 2 years 1899-1912 (per 1000) in France

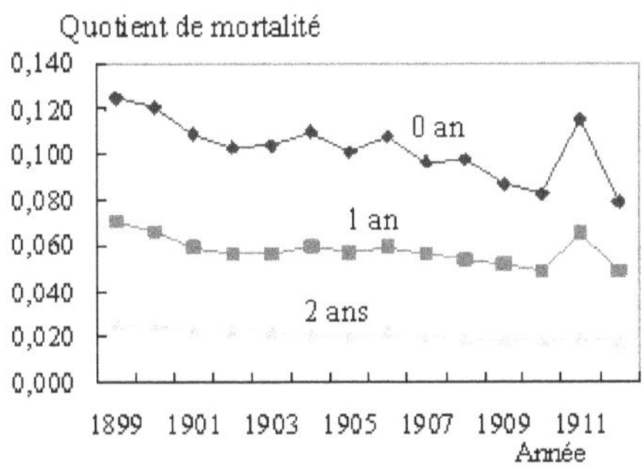

Source: Rollet, 'La canicule'.

Table 2. Probabilities of deaths at 0, 1 and 2 year olds, both sexes 1899-1910 (‰)

Year	Age (in years)		
	Under 1	1 year	2 years
1899-1900	122.75	68.30	25.06
1901-1905	105.37	57.88	21.52
1906-1910	94.34	54.24	19.46

Source : Rollet, 'La canicule'.

42 Strauss, P. *La croisade sanitaire*. Paris, Bibliothèque-Charpentier, 1902.

43 Rollet, C. 'La canicule de 1911. Réalités démographiques, observations médicales et réactions politiques', in *Hommage à Jacques Vallin*, Paris, Ined, 2009.

The virtues of water, sunshine and fresh air: under medical control (1914-1940)

After World War One the *Statistique générale de la France* re-classified infantile deaths to the department of birth and the parents' home, thus allowing a more accurate calculation of infant mortality rates.[44] As a result those departments which sent out children for fostering had significant increases: for the years 1921 and 1922 averaging 28 per cent in the department of the Seine (nearly one-quarter of whom actually died in other departments) and over 18 per cent in the Rhône. Infant mortality rates in the fostering departments decreased correspondingly, in 1920 by 31 per cent in Eure-et-Loir, by 34 per cent in Nièvre and 25 per cent in the Ardèche. Thus, the areas of high mortality were more clearly revealed: the industrial departments of Normandy, the East and North of France and a large region south of the Central Mountains and Provence recorded rates exceeding 90 per 1,000. In contrast western, south-western and central France were regions of lower infant mortality (Table 3).

Table 3. Infant mortality rates according to place of birth, 1920-1924 (per 1,000)

Highest rates		**Lowest rates**	
Seine-Inférieure	127	Creuse	63
Bouches-du-Rhône	125	Indre	63
Seine	122	Nièvre	64
Calvados	115	Landes	65
Ille-et-Vilaine	115	Cher	65
Rhône	112	Vienne	68
Moselle	112	Deux-Sèvres	71
Lot	110	Allier	71
Corse	110	Cher	73
Haute-Loire	109	Vendée	74

Source: SGF, 1928.

At this time interest in rural life, characterised by fresh air, sunshine and good soil, was increasing, with some physicians adopting Rousseau's ideas and adding some scientific dimensions. The older health mentality was now offered as a solution for improving the health status of the whole French population. Many diseases resulting in infant deaths, such as typhoid fever, diarrhoea or infantile cholera had been traced to polluted water and, along with the value of pure water, the role of sunlight was now emphasised in the prevention of rickets and tuberculosis. Since the countryside as opposed to towns had such resources, the first step needed was to make sure that urban children had access to these benefits.

---

44 Statistique générale de la France, *Statistique du mouvement de la population*, Nouvelle série, tome IV, Annexes 1920 à 1924, Paris, 1928, CI et CV.

In Switzerland, Doctor Rollier had developed the concept of 'School in the Sunshine' as a means of preventing tuberculosis. His book, published in 1914, shows beautiful colour photographs of naked children conducting their various activities in the sunshine: schooling, gymnastics, lunches, naps etc.[45] Some French physicians had already begun to place infants from tuberculosis-affected families in rural foster homes and a new institution, the 'Oeuvre du Placement familial des Tout-Petits' was established in 1921 to develop these arrangements for very young infants. Under the direction of Doctors Léon Bernard and Robert Debré, it managed seven centres of foster families, caring for 215 children in the Sologne region. Similar arrangements were made in Lyon by Doctor Mouriquand, whereby children lived in foster families in a village of the department of Isère until they were eighteen months old. From 1924 to 1932, 210 babies were placed in this manner but these numbers were small and systematic use of the BCG vaccine, also developed in 1921, protected many more children, with 4,328 vaccinated in 1925 but 210,668 in 1935.[46] For older children, Armand-Delille had established an open-air school in Monnetier, Savoie in 1921, with lessons given outside in the best place under the trees.[47]

Here was the reactivating of a very old method, the placing in a foster family in the countryside, but with the considerable difference that these institutions were directly controlled by specialists in tuberculosis; families were carefully chosen; medical control was strict and babies and families were visited frequently. In effect, children were placed in 'bringing-up centres' in medically and morally-approved environments. Mrs Gonse-Boas, who created the 'Nouvelle étoile des enfants de France' in 1913 explained that families with nice homes and few children were best. The woman chosen needed to be neat and tidy and ready scrupulously to keep the rules, with the foster family given the equipment necessary: bed, steriliser, thermometer, tub, and even sterilised milk provided daily by the nurse.[48] Each centre was placed under the control of a physician and a health visitor. Rare in southern areas, these centres were mainly set up in departments like Oise, Seine-et-Oise, Nord, Loir-et-Cher, Seine-et-Marne, Eure

---

45 Rollier, A. *La cure de soleil*, Paris, Baillière et fils et Constant Tarin, 1914. In 1944, he presented his forty- year experience in heliotherapy especially at the School of Leysin for the children of Lausanne. See Heller, G., 'La cure intensive d'hygiène en Suisse. Les écoles de plein air au début du XXe siècle', in Châtelet, A. M ; Lerch, D. ; Luc, J.-N, *L'école de plein air. Une expérience pédagogique et architecturale dans l'Europe du XXe siècle*, Focales, Editions Recherches, 2003, 211-221.

46 Rollet, *La politique à l'égard*, 208.

47 Coffin, J.-C. 'Paul-Félix Armand-Delille (1874-1964). Vertu thérapeutique du milieu et action sociale en faveur de l'enfance', in Châtelet, Lerch and Luc, *L'école de plein air...*, 222-229.

48 Gonse-Boas (Mme), 'Dispensaires d'hygiène infantile et centres d'élevage', *Revue d'hygiène*, 1921, 1036.

and Orne. Sixty centres were working in 1930; still few considering that about 40,000 children were in foster families in France at that time. Ironically, the reticence of health visitors to stay in the countryside was seen as one of the obstacles to the proliferation of these centres.

By now the returning popularity of the countryside and its virtues was spreading in all directions. Heliotropism, hydrotherapy and aerotherapy were fashionable, judging by the experiences of the various departments and indeed throughout Europe. *L'Illustration's* report in 1931 on the kinder garden set up by the town of Aubervilliers in Dugny (Seine-et-Oise) is representative, describing how all activities took place outdoors, including naps in the shade of the trees, sunbathing (naked children, bellies to the ground, heads protected by linen hats), meals, lessons, practical work and showers. Doctor Lemière's photographs aptly depict the belief in sunlight, fresh air, space as having properties able to 'regenerate these two hundred tiny tots preserved from the smog of the suburbs'.[49]

Ecole maternelle at Dugny (near Paris), 1931: the class

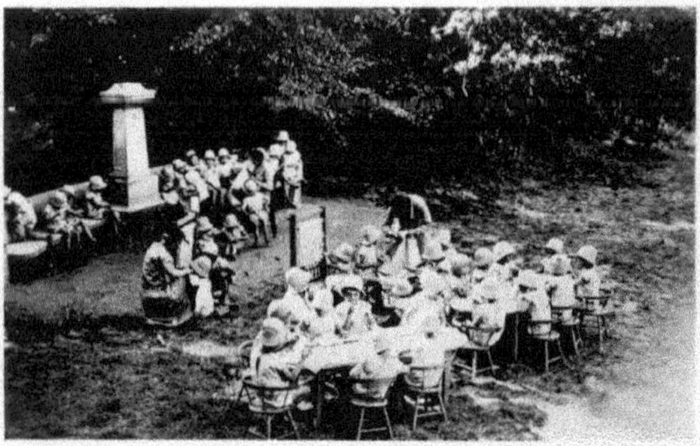

Ecole maternelle at Dugny (near Paris), 1931: the nap

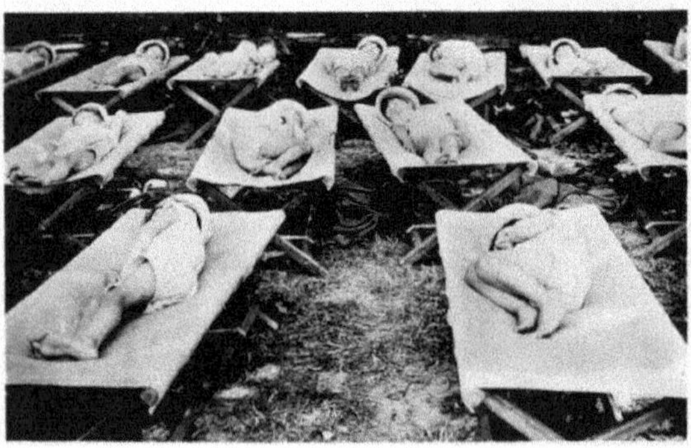

Children were recruited by doctors, a dozen per school, and boarded for three months, being entirely cared for by a team composed of a headmistress, two mistresses, a school nurse and five assistants.[50] Epidemics were rare because children were vaccinated

49 'Un paradis pour enfants', *L'Illustration*, n° 4612, 25 juillet 1931, 464.

50 'L'Ecole de plein air d'Aubervilliers à Dugny (Seine)', in *Congrès international pour la protection de l'enfance*, Comité national de l'enfance, 1933, LXVII-LXXIX.

before their stay. The authors of *Open-Air Schools,* describing such institutions all over Europe, argued that, beyond the sanitary aim, open-air schools represented an innovative and pedagogic project. This ensured not just healthy bodies, but a broadening of the mind beyond burdensome school programmes and stereotyped knowledge so that individual growth and active involvement replaced the mechanisms of passive apprenticeship. Such ideals corresponded to the New School, more developed in France, the Netherlands and Sweden than elsewhere.

Another significant example, provided by Paul Carton, former hospital physician in Paris, then doctor in the Brévannes hospital (Seine-et-Oise), had strong eugenicist overtones.[51] A prime objective was to 'rebuild a strong and healthy race' and similarly, 'we have to come back to the road of nature and reason in a world threatened by false science which leads to a hedonistic lifestyle and its consequences', 'depopulation' and 'degeneration'. He opposed the 'misuse' of medicine and vaccination, seen as 'weakening the race', seeking a return to natural laws, a more natural diet, and an emphasis upon health as a prerogative obtained through effort and merit. He utilised the sun-cure, carefully surveyed, with gymnastics and games allowing the child to reinforce his natural defences and grow harmoniously. His methods were to be adapted to each age and situation (sickness or health), guarding against the excesses of naturism seen in Germany and the over-control evident in the keeping of a personal health record, instituted in 1934 in France.[52] Such terminology featured throughout inter-war Europe, compounded by international conflicts and the post-1929 economic crisis, as issues of race and other 'threats' to regeneration were 'scientifically' determined. The tonality of the discourse was far different from that of the pre-war years, as 'quality' began to compete with quantity.

However, these initiatives still favoured the needs of the urban population and children under public welfare, rather than those of rural families. During the Paris Conference on Child Welfare in 1933, discussion concerning practical education for mothers to guard against infantile mortality included the rural population specifically. Léonie Gillet revealed that, whereas infant mortality in 1932 was 70 per 1,000 in the city of Lyon, in the rural municipalities of the department of Rhône, it varied between 100 and 170 per 1,000. [53] The countryside had been neglected and her experience in social work had made her familiar

51 Carton, P. *La cure de soleil et d'exercices chez les enfants*, Docteur Paul Carton, 1935, 1-6.

52 Ross, C. *Naked Germany. Health, Race and the Nation*, Berg, 2005. Controls in France began in 1935 for babies in care and 1937 for all babies. See: Rollet, C. *Les carnets de santé des enfants*, Paris, La Dispute, 2008.

53 Mme Edmond Gillet, 'Un essai d'éducation des mères à la campagne', *Congrès international pour la protection de l'enfance*, Comité national de l'enfance, 1933, 195-203.

with the hard struggle against infant mortality in rural areas. Problems of distance and isolation meant that the education of rural mothers required new means, notably motor-cars and films.

The insurance and savings bank of the department, in connection with the department council, had provided a bus and mobile facilities to assist mothers and children. From December, 1932, this measure allowed the transportation of 'baby weighing to the door of the most isolated home' and offered training for young girls and young mothers. The hygiene puericulture demonstration concerned food, bandages, clothing, poultices and cupping glasses, hygiene of the sick, healthcare for pregnant women and new-born babies, preparation of feeding bottles, layette, cradle, etc. Such services suited everyone: the nurse could stay for a few days to look after a sick child; elsewhere, the training session ended with a film; while village children were given a check-up thanks to the 'little baby bus'. Visiting nurses adapted to rural women, taking care that 'they are uncomplicated, approachable, always cheerful, and they don't impose themselves. Their advice is wise, practical, and always easy to apply and they don't ask the impossible. …They are already very popular in the municipality' according to one local Mayor.[54] Though a great benefit, the system of ambulatory consultations was incomplete until every county had a polyvalent nurse equipped with adequate means of transportation and more health visitors had the use of motor-cars rather than bicycles to increase their mobility.

The little baby bus (L'ambulance des tout-petits)

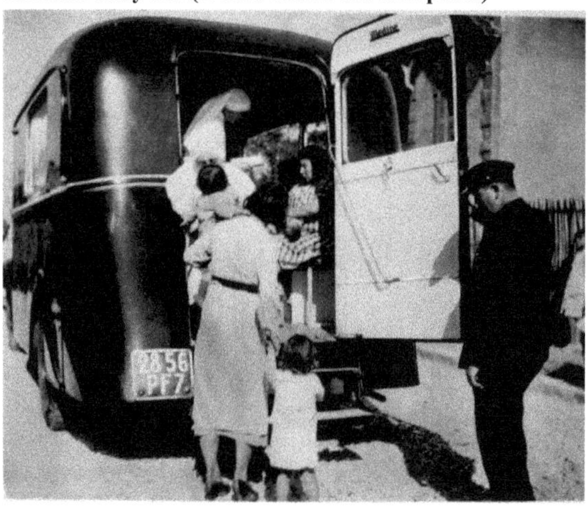

Source: *Le visage de l'enfance,* 1937

M.A. Eynard, Inspector of Public Welfare in the same department, also discussed the demographic deficit in the countryside, voicing the need to

> 'create an organization capable of giving the practical education which is lacking at present to mothers from the countryside. They have never learnt the elementary

54 Letter April 25th, 1933 cited in Gillet, 1933.

> principles of infant hygiene and of baby feeding. They keep in mind the empirical methods of their grandmothers which they often practice in spite of the opinions of medical doctors and nurses ... Old prejudice and routines have not yet completely disappeared'. [55]

He emphasised the paradox of rural excess-mortality, 'although fresh air, sunlight and good milk should ensure the best chances of survival to the new-born babies'. Like Mme Gillet, he recommended home visits by health visitors and puericulture training for young schoolgirls and planned a county dispensary under the auspices of a medical doctor specialised in puericulture. Though such testimony indicated the ongoing process of 'acculturation', more than half a century had passed before rural populations – even those resistant, could access new scientific knowledge and have their own resources recognised.

In the department of Gironde, it was noted that the law on social insurance gave rise to a fresh interest in consultations for pregnant women and babies, 'especially in the countryside', giving weight to the saying 'prevention is better than cure'.[56] Meanwhile the Secretary General of the Feminist Group of Auch, commissioned by the National Council of French Women, discussed the return of young middle class women to the countryside. The tone was both down-to-earth and idyllic, centred upon proposals that young women from a modest background and needing full-time work, might settle in the countryside on small farms of six to eight hectares, starting a family and bringing up children. Surrounded by their parents' love, these children would grow up 'good-looking and healthy as they run through the fields and breathe in the fresh air'! Evidently one lady was planning to organise in her

The health visitor and the mother or the foster mother

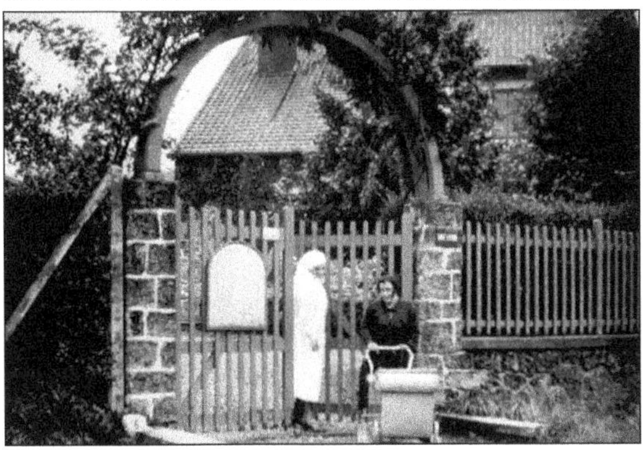

Source: *Le visage de l'enfance,* 1937

55 Eynard, M. A. 'Etat d'instruction des mères et nourrices de la campagne en matière d'hygiène infantile. Comment et par qui peut-on éduquer ?', *Congrès...*, 205-208.

56 Docteur Rocaz, 'Assurances sociales et éducation technique des mères ', *Congrès...*, 225-227.

castle in Monroussin, the practical rural knowledge needed for training these women, with the farms bought with the help of the State.[57]

Between the two World Wars, mutual insurance tried to support mothers with the establishment of small rural maternity clinics, a project then considered as 'the realization of the future for the protection of motherhood'. Equipped to cater for around twenty women, they were also used for prenatal consultations and women stayed there for two to three weeks.[58] The provision for the rural population of equipments previously reserved for towns was an indicator of the entrance of the rural world into modernity, though the installation of running water, gas and electricity, which was to greatly facilitate the work of the housewife, would appear later.

The prominent actor in supporting rural as well as urban populations was the visiting nurse for social hygiene, an exclusively feminine, professional body, created in 1924 by Paul Strauss, the Minister of Hygiene. Specialising in the prevention of tuberculosis and infant mortality and in educating mothers, they came to the families' homes. Under the auspices of a medical doctor, they followed his instructions by advising the mothers, recommending solutions to improve living conditions, food and basic rules of hygiene. They had some equipment but worked as mediators between the doctors, responsible for the people's health, and the families.[59] In France, they were controlled by the medical corporation.

Conclusion

Thus the inversion of the perspective from the 1860's and the inter-war period was complete: the countryside, previously under-equipped, began to benefit from a programme of economic and medico-social development. Its integration into the national territory was reinforced and its assets – notably the living conditions from which the rural and the urban population was able to benefit – were at last realised. These assets were known but were now more attainable, because of scientific knowledge and the process of universalisation at work. Babies from countryside and from cities, (and not only nurslings), might now benefit from these resources. The symbol of the unification of the territory as far as infant mortality is concerned was seen in the publishing in 1939 of the first official health file covering all children, rural or urban, and assisted or not.

---

57 Mme Franck Doizan, 'Le retour à la campagne des jeunes femmes de la petite bourgeoisie. Son importance au point de vue de la mère et de l'enfant', *Congrès*..., 373-377.

58 Gros, F.-L., 'La puériculture d'aujourd'hui', in *Le visage de l'enfance*, Paris, 1937, 101-102. F.-Louise Gros is administrative assistant of the Comité national de l'enfance, member of the High Council of Public Welfare (Conseil supérieur de l'Assistance publique).

59 Their role was subsumed within the body of social workers from 1938.

Nevertheless, the romantic picture of a healthy life in the countryside was typical of the Vichy ideology, evident in the illustrations of a book on puericulture published by the National Committee for Infancy in 1943.[60] The artist André Marty skillfully depicted this utopian idea of the education of children far from the city and industries: just as the farmer kept an eye on the growth of his crops, the mother was entirely devoted to the care of her children, applying the advice of the child specialist and the nurse. Thus puericulture is seen in this book in its whole etymological dimension: the art of rearing, of taking care of children, from the latin words, *puer* and *colo, colis, colere*. But the actual social and economic background of the French country was completely forgotten in this kind of representation and new post-war legislation sought to re-equilibrate the policy both toward countryside and cities, ensuring equality in rights between families and children.[61]

60 Comité national de l'enfance, *Problèmes et aspects de la puériculture moderne*, Paris, 1943.

61 Norvez, A. *De la naissance à l'école. Santé, modes de garde et préscolarité dans la France contemporaine*, Paris, Ined/Puf, 1990, 79-80.

SERVING THE COUNTRYSIDE IN TIMES OF CRISIS: NORWAY 1912-1940

Astri Andresen and Teemu Ryymin

In many European countries the early twentieth century witnessed growing state involvement in the health and welfare of the population, as demonstrated in previous chapters. At the same time self-help and local autonomy continued to be important. The process and consequently the relationship between local and central, or private and public, took on varying shapes in various European countries. It contributed in producing quite different post-war welfare systems, from the corporatist welfare regimes in southern Europe to the social democratic and universalistic ones in the Scandinavian countries.[1] In Norway and other Nordic countries, rural interests played a major role in giving the welfare state its particular form based upon universality: in the early twentieth century out of rural strength, in 1945 out of conceived weaknesses.[2]

Health policies played a vital role and in this paper we argue the following points. First, that the early twentieth-century Norwegian health care system sought to create better and more equal access to health services; between social classes, urban and rural societies, and different regions. Judged by growing numbers of medical officers of health (MosH), medical institutions and their improved distribution, the system succeeded in creating equality in this sense. In fact, Norwegian health policies in this period were so successful that features not anticipated by central authorities emerged, notably more widespread demand for 'the doctor', many more medical institutions and far greater patient numbers within these. Second, the basic tenets of the health care system, established by the 1900 Tuberculosis Act, the 1909 Sickness Insurance Act and the 1912 Public Medical Services Act, were maintained throughout the inter-war period, despite growing economic problems, governmental cut-backs and increased antagonism between central and peripheral districts. Even so, equality in health services was given a prominent place on the political agenda in 1945 and a third point, as we have argued elsewhere, was that, after a generation of 'equalisation',

1 Esping-Andersen, G. *The three worlds of Welfare Capitalism*, Princeton, Princeton University Press, 1991, 25-29. Cf. also Christiansen, N.F.; Petersen, K.; Edling, N.; Haave, P. (eds.) *The Nordic Model of Welfare. A Historical Reappraisal*, Copenhagen, Museum Tusculanum Press, 2006.

2 Christiansen et al., *The Nordic Model*, 17-20.

understandings of what 'equality' and 'access to health services' actually meant had been transformed.[3]

It is often postulated that welfare policies are particularly path-dependant; that traditions play an important role in identifying problems and appropriate solutions.[4] One might for example consider the important long-term role of the Catholic Church in relief as decisive in the place it attained in southern European welfare regimes after World War Two. But at the same time welfare is an arena for major changes and mind-sets might be altered by the shock of war, as Steve King and John Stewart have noted, but also in more peaceful times.[5] The changing mind-set that we point to here is the seemingly newborn faith in what physicians and medical institutions could do, both in public health and curative practices, that developed among ordinary people in Norway in the two decades after 1900. When it comes to faith in medical practitioners per se, our impression is that the population in Norway – or the Nordic countries – was a late-comer compared to other European populations. We do notice, however, W. F. Bynum's observation that, 'Whether the patient of 1914 would have had more confidence in the doctor than his grandparents would have had in theirs is another matter'.[6] Where faith in medical institutions is concerned, as in preparedness to become a hospital patient and expectation of a successful outcome, we find Norway more or less 'in line' with other nations, for example America between 1900 and 1930, where hospitals were 'praised as monuments to humanity and science.'[7] The important question is why this happened in those years. Was it simply that more hospitals and medical practitioners became available and that they satisfied growing needs? Or was the main reason, as is often suggested, that the period 1900-1930 saw a general increase in both political and public trust in science? [8] And if so, did this reflect fundamental changes in how doctors themselves thought about medical institutions?

Before developing our three points, a few comments on topography, population and health are called for, since these inform the accessibility and meaning of health care, as also demonstrated in particular by Paola M. Melis and Lucia

---

3 Ryymin, T. and Andresen, A. 'Effecting equality: Norwegian Health Policy in Finnmark, 1945-1970s', *Acta Borealia*, 26:1, 2009, 96 – 114.

4 Christiansen et al., *The Nordic Model*, 16.

5 King, S. and Stewart, J. (eds.) *Welfare peripheries. The Development of Welfare States in Nineteenth and Twentieth Century Europe*, Bern, Peter Lang, 2007.

6 Bynum, W. F. *Science and the Practice of Medicine in the Nineteenth Century*, Cambridge, Cambridge University Press, 1994, 177.

7 Risse, G.B. *Mending Bodies, Saving Souls. A History of Hospitals*, New York/Oxford, Oxford University Press, 1999, 468.

8 Risse, *Mending Bodies*, 463-512. Borowy, I. and Gruner, W.D. (eds.) *Facing Illness in Troubled Times*, Frankfurt am Main, Peter Lang, 2005, 2-5.

Pozzi and Tore Grønlie's chapters in this volume. One might be led to believe that Norway is the only country in Europe with a geography and topography that – in some districts – made communication and access to health care very difficult and expensive. That is of course not the case; the topography and distances in the Alps, the north of Scotland, the Pyrenees, Sardinia and many other areas and regions have also surely posed severe challenges to the respective medical authorities.

Allowing such points, the distances involved in some Norwegian regions were huge and communications were difficult and slow. In 1913 for example, to get the doctor from his residence to the inland village of Kautokeino in Finnmark might take seven or eight days.[9] Norway was also an overwhelmingly rural country and among the most sparsely populated in Europe. Both in 1900 and 1946 28 per cent of the population lived in towns.[10] Since a town was defined according to formal status, Norwegian censuses established a category in between the rural and the urban, namely 'population agglomerations'. That part of the population living in such agglomerations increased from 7.7 per cent in 1900 to 22.1 per cent in 1946.[11] Agglomerations were in some cases similar to towns, sometimes suburban areas, yet they could also be very small: for 1900-1910 the defining criteria were at least 20 houses and 200 inhabitants; for 1920-1946, 20 houses and at least 100 inhabitants.[12] Thus, allowing 'agglomerations', it remains safe to say that the rural character of Norway continued throughout the period under investigation. Infant mortality was lower in rural districts than in towns until the period 1936-1940, when the rural rate was 39.6 per 1,000 births and the urban one 38.5 per 1,000. In 1901-1905, it had been 70.4 per 1,000 in rural districts and 103.3 per 1,000 in towns so, obviously, the towns experienced a faster decrease than the countryside.[13] Using infant mortality as an indicator of general health status, urban environments were worse off than rural until the 1930s but, when the tables turned, the advantage to the towns was very small.

---

9 Stortingets forhandlinger (the parliamentary debate) 1913, 30 June, 2111.

10 Backer, J. *Dødeligheten og dens årsaker i Norge 1856-1955*, Samfunnsøkonomiske studier nr. 10. Oslo, Statistisk sentralbyrå, 1961, 24.

11 Backer, *Dødeligheten*, 24.

12 Norges officielle statistikk Fjerde Række nr. 52. Folketellingen i Kongeriget Norge 3 December 1900 første hefte. Kristiania, Det Statistiske Centralbureau, 1902, 149; Norges officielle statistik V. 170. Folketællingen i Norge 1 December 1910 første hefte. Det statistiske Centralbyrå. Kristiania, Aschehoug & Co. 1912, 154; Norges offisielle statistikk VII. 39. Folketellingen i Norge 1. desember 1920 første hefte. Det statistiske Centralbyrå. Kristiania, H. Aschehoug & Co, 1922, 164; Norges offisielle statistikk. VIII. 182. Folketellingen i Norge 1 desember 1930 første hefte. Det Statistiske centralbyrå. Oslo, Aschehoug & Co, 1932, 146; Norges offisielle statistikk XI. 2. Folketellingen i Norge 3. desember 1946 første hefte. Statistisk Sentralbyrå. Oslo, H. Aschehoug & Co, 1950, 117.

13 Backer, *Dødeligheten*, 60.

Standardised rates for general mortality also revealed only minor differences between rural and urban societies, with the exception of male town-dwellers who experienced higher rates than women and their rural counterparts.[14]

These figures indicate that no dramatic, systematic inequality of health existed between rural and urban societies in the first half of the twentieth century. Yet they hide huge regional differences, particularly with regard to infant mortality, as Table 1 illustrates for the three northernmost counties in the country, compared to the national average.

Table 1. Regional infant mortality per 1,000 live births: Northern Norway and Norwegian average 1911-1945

Year	Nordland county	Troms county	Finnmark county	Norway (av.)
1911-15	60	72	129	66
1921-25	54	66	112	52
1931-35	43	62	92	45
1941-45	40	54	84	37

Source: Balsvik, R. R. and Drake, M. 'Menneskene i Nord-Norge fra istid til nåtid – fra vogge til grav', in Drivenes, E.-A. (ed.) *Nordnorsk kulturhistorie bd. 1. Det gjenstridige landet*, Oslo, Gyldendal norsk forlag, 1994, 128.

Even between neighbouring counties the differences were marked, Nordland county having rates below the national average, whereas the Finnmark rates were twice as high.

The establishment of a new health care system

Between 1900 and 1912 three significant Acts pertaining to health care were approved in the Norwegian Parliament. In 1900, Norway passed the first national Tuberculosis Act in the world, followed by the 1909 Sickness Insurance Act and a new Public Medical Services Act in 1912. Each act addressed separate health and welfare issues but together they established a dynamic system of health care provision which stimulated the building of health institutions and enhanced the dispersal of medical services to steadily increasing numbers of Norwegian citizens, regardless of their abode. Moreover such legislation reflected growing state involvement in the regulation of spheres of life with relevance to illness and health. From the late 1880s areas ranging from schools to the inspection of factories and the control of cemeteries were all regulated through national Acts. While many of the new laws dictated how different issues were to be dealt with locally, others left the local municipalities in charge of realising the law-givers' intentions. Overall, such legislation provided a legal and fiscal framework for

14 Backer, *Dødeligheten*, 48.

the municipalities to work within, thereby creating a system characteristic of the self-help-orientated social policies of the period.[15]

In the rural health care context the Tuberculosis Act and the Sickness Insurance Act provided particularly important impulses to institution building in the countryside, while the Public Medical Services Act addressed the organisation of public health work and improved access to medical treatment; each personified in the state medical officer of health (MosH).[16]

Let us briefly examine the effects of these Acts, beginning with the MosH. The 1912 Public Medical Services Act increased dramatically the number of medical districts in Norway from 161 to 372.[17] Similarly, according to the national budget, there were 156 state MosH in 1912 and 367 by 1923.[18] Not unsurprisingly, physicians were in great demand and by the end of World War One, it was very difficult to recruit to the most strenuous and least lucrative positions in peripheral Norway.[19] Nevertheless the 1912 Act was largely implemented in the early 1920s which, among other developments, contributed to lower inhabitants per doctor ratios. These fell from 2,012 persons per doctor in 1910 to 1,591 per doctor in 1930 and to 1,265 per doctor in 1940.[20] Most of the post-1912 state MosH were district medical officers serving in rural communities, so it appears that the latter benefited particularly, even though great differentials remained regarding rural health services.[21]

In the early 1920s the implementation of the 1912 Act benefited from the approaching crisis that reduced the private market for medical services and sustained the increase in the number of medical applicants. Moreover it was well supported by authorities and inhabitants in rural Norway. For example, even if some municipalities felt compelled by central authorities to build new dwellings for new medical officers, they gladly did so in order to get a doctor and most

---

15 Cf. Hovland, E. 'Grotid og glanstid. 1837-1920', in Næss, H.E. et al. (eds.) *Folkestyre i by og bygd. Norske kommuner gjennom 150 år*, Oslo/Bergen/Stavanger/Tromsø, Universitetsforlaget, 1987: 114-117, 127-136; Angell, S.I. *Den svenske modellen og det norske systemet. Tilhøvet mellom modernisering og identitetsdanning i Sverige og Norge ved overgangen til det 20. hundreåret*, Oslo, Det norske Samlaget, 2002, 152-208.

16 Schiøtz. A. *Det offentlige helsevesen i Norge 1603-2003, Folkets helse – landets styrke 1850-2003*, Oslo, Universitetsforlaget, 2003, 151-53.

17 Schiøtz, *Det offentlige helsevesen*, 152.

18 St. prp. Nr. 1. Hovedpost VI kap. 10, title 1-2 (1912), 1; St. prp. Nr. 1. Hovedpost VII B kap. 5 (1924), 1.

19 The state Director of Medicine in *Tidsskrift for Den norske lægeforening, 37* (1917), 878. Also Stortingets forhandlinger (the parliamentary debate), 30th March 1917, 706 – 721.

20 Schiøtz, A. *Doktoren. Distriktslegenes historie 1900-1984*, Oslo, Pax Forlag A/S, 2003, 456 (Table 2).

21 Schiøtz, *Doktoren*, 455 (Table 1).

municipalities were enthusiastic and financially respondent to the call from central authorities to act.[22]

Not only were the MosH very welcome in rural Norway but medical institutions were also built in great numbers in the countryside in the 1910s and 1920s. This was made possible through several Acts pertaining to health care. The 1909 Sickness Insurance Act (*syketrygden*), passed after years of political strife and conflict, sought – like the 1912 Act on State medical officers – to enhance and make equitable popular access to health services.[23] The Sickness Insurance Act made membership in municipal health insurance societies (*sykekasse*) mandatory for employees with salaries under a certain limit. The insurance premium was divided between the state contributing 20 per cent, municipality and employer paying ten per cent each, and the insured were to pay 60 per cent themselves. If society members or their spouses or children fell ill, their loss of income would be compensated, with medical treatment and some assistance paid for a limited period of time. Crucially members' stays in medical institutions would also be paid for, with hospital costs partly reimbursed through insurance premiums and public funds. This created a secure source of funding for health institutions, making it more feasible for local communities to establish their own.[24] The number of people insured rose from 330,000 in 1912 to 592,722 in 1926, and reached over one million – or 65 per cent of the work force in the 15-70 age range – in 1938, as salary limits were adjusted and some self-employed groups such as fishermen and sailors were included. It was also possible to join voluntarily: by 1926, 12.6 per cent (approximately 75,000 individuals) of the local health insurance society members were enrolled voluntarily, and in 1938 they numbered 178,000.[25]

The system of municipal health insurance societies – as opposed to a single national insurance society, which had been originally suggested by the Parliamentary commission first launching the issue in 1895 – was in part a result of

---

22 Stortingets forhandlinger (Parliamentary debate), 17th April 1923, 892-93.

23 Bjørnson, Ø.; Haavet, I.E. *Langsomt ble landet et velferdssamfunn. Trygdens historie 1894-1994*, Oslo, Ad Notam Gyldendal, 1994, 55-79.

24 Stene-Larsen, G. 'Home Visits or Hospital Beds?' in Larsen Ø. (ed.) *The Shaping of a Profession. Physicians in Norway, Past and Present*, Canton, Mass., Science History Publications, 1996, 361; Hansen, F.H. 'Sykehusstruktur i historisk perspektiv', in Hansen, F.H. (ed.) *SAMDATA Sykehus Rapport. Sykehusstruktur i endring. De lange linjer og utviklingen siste tiår*, Trondheim, SINTEF Unimed NIS SAMDATA/Kommuneforlaget, 2001, 36-37.

25 Ot.prp. nr. 46 (1928) *Om å utferdige en lov om endringer i lov om sykeforsikring av 6. august 1915 med tilleggslover*. Appendix 1: *Innstilling fra Den departementale sykeforsikringskomité av 1927*, 7 (Table 3); Bjørnson and Haavet, *Langsomt ble landet et velferdssamfunn*, 55-79.

the intervention by rural interests during the prolonged Parliamentary discussions and investigations into the matter between 1900-1909. A national insurance society that would treat both urban and rural areas alike was feared to lead to a transfer of funds from the perceivably healthier rural population to the urban working class. The municipal solution agreed upon in 1909, with differentiated premiums based on the risk of illness among different occupations, was to hinder this – the end result being lower premiums for servants and other rural workers compared with urban workers.[26]

The importance of the 1909 Sickness Insurance Act for institution building has been noted on several occasions. However, analysis of the historical growth of medical institutions in Norway has often focused on somatic hospitals, usually privileged as the most important in accordance with the role they gained in Norwegian health policies particularly after World War Two. However, other early twentieth-century institutions were also important components in the health care system, particularly in the rural context. For instance, the 1900 Tuberculosis Act had already established a mechanism of economic redistribution from the public to health institutions similar to that established under the 1909 Act. The Tuberculosis Act stated that the costs of patients committed by local Health Boards to hospitals or other institutions would be paid for by the state, the county and the patient's municipality, according to a partial funding scheme which secured TB institutions a steady income of public money. State authorities also encouraged private organisations to establish such institutions, in cooperation with county and municipal administrations. Many early twentieth-century doctors believed that small, widely dispersed institutions in the countryside were most desirable, particularly in the fight against tuberculosis.[27]

This system of public-private institution funding and building, primarily established to create greater economic equality in times of illness and to ensure that the most widespread infectious disease of the time would be curtailed in all parts of the country, proved to be a forceful impetus for private entrepreneurship. It also stimulated what has been termed 'welfare localism' for, given a degree of financial security, local communities and private actors embarked on a huge project of institution building.[28] Between 1900 and 1940, a new type of

---

26 Bjørnson and Haavet, *Langsomt ble landet et velferdssamfunn*, 65-69.

27 *Tidsskrift for Den norske lægeforening*, 24 (1904), 603; cf. Ryymin, T. *Smitte, språk og kultur. Tuberkulosearbeidet i Finnmark 1900-1960*, Oslo, Scandinavian Academic Press/Spartacus, 2009.

28 On the system of private-public cooperation, see Seip, A.-L. 'Velferdskommunen og velferdstrekanten – et tilbakeblikk', in Nagel, A.-H. (ed.) *Velferdskommunen. Kommunenes rolle i utviklingen av velferdsstaten*, Bergen, Alma Mater, 1991, 24-42; Martinsen, K. *Omsorg, sykepleie og medisin. Historisk-filosofiske essays*, Oslo, TANO, 1989, 131. On welfare localism, see Grønlie, T. 'Norwegian General Hospitals, 1970-

tuberculosis nursing home, catering for patients with end-stage pulmonary tuberculosis, was established, and numerous general or somatic hospitals were built.[29] Many of these were rather small and some 222 of the 400 medical institutions were located in the countryside in 1940.[30] Excepting the counties of Eastern and Western Agder in Southern Norway, which had no rural institutions at all in 1940, it appears that until then the greatest numerical growth of medical institutions took place in rural Norway. Thus, smaller hospitals and other medical institutions not only became 'Main Street's civic pride', but also the pride of many rural municipalities.[31] Still, compared with the spatial dispersion of the general population, there existed an urban bias regarding the location of medical institutions. In 1946, only about 28 per cent of the population in Norway resided in towns, while in 1940 44.5 per cent of all medical institutions were located there, although many general hospitals (as Tore Grønlie demonstrates below) also served the surrounding rural areas.

The majority of the Norwegian rural medical institutions in 1940 were small tuberculosis nursing homes or facilities combining tuberculosis and general hospital beds. Only 15 of the 52 rural general hospitals had special wards for surgical or internal (*indremedisinske*) cases. Most of the small general cottage hospitals (*bygdesykehus*) were non-specified, offering services for accident cases, acute infections, minor surgery and observation.[32] The growth of the rural health institutions was mainly a result of local initiatives and responses to perceived problems, with central blessing and funding secured through the health insurance system and/or the TB act but without central planning. Hospitals in urban areas also flourished with the financial security provided by the 1909 Act but they all benefited from charges to rural patients that were covered by local health insurance societies.

It may thus be claimed that the system established in the early 1900s was a great success. Further, it worked alongside and collaboratively with the system of MosH who might attend patients at the tuberculosis home or cottage hospital or decide to hospitalise a patient in the first place. The MosH was in any case also responsible for the treatment of the sick poor, many of whom resided in such institutions.

2002: County Ownership – An Interlude between Welfare Localism and State Direction', *Medical History, 50* (2006), 192.

29 Cf. Bu, S. *Sykehusene i Norge*. Chr. Gundersens boktrykkeri, Oslo, 1941.

30 The following is based on information on number and location of Norwegian medical institutions in Bu, *Sykehusene*.

31 Risse, *Mending bodies*, 463,

32 Cf. Bu, *Sykehusene*, 64, 78.

Economic crisis and restructuring

Economic crisis was a permanent feature of Norwegian society during most of the 1920s and first half of the 1930s, affecting the established health care system as the state attempted to reduce costs.[33] Committees to cut state spending were set up in 1923, 1927 and in 1932 and reductions in the numbers of medical districts and of MosH were proposed. It was argued, for example, that motor boats, roads and cars as modern means of communication were not common when the 1912 Act was passed, but these now justified 143 fewer state MosH. [34] To offset this reduction in part, municipalities would be financially supported to hire less expensive community doctors to supplement the remaining state MosH.

However, the Parliament rejected these proposals on three main grounds. First, the transport revolution had not reached all regions, particularly not Northern and Western Norway, and access to health care was still an issue. In fact, seldom were the differences between the central regions of Eastern Norway and the peripheral west and north so strongly emphasised. Moreover, the public health tasks had expanded vastly since 1912, as had popular expectations of medical assistance and actual use of doctors. Third, the present good situation regarding public and individual health might deteriorate to pre-1912 conditions, 'leaving us once more with lice and who knows what ugly things'.[35] Indeed several members of parliament emphasised that the 1912 Act in particular had successfully brought equality to rural populations, which the state should maintain even during times of deep economic crisis.

A fundamental reason for the resistance against the proposed cuts may be found in changed perceptions of the necessity of medical services provided by doctors. In the 1910s, an argument for employing medical officers was that the population had grown accustomed to using them.[36] In the 1930s, however, having access to the doctor was now seen as a matter of life and death.[37] This was the main reason why 'the doctor' became a trusted figure, demonstrably the 'mediator' between life and death. Not unsurprisingly, accidents and difficult and life-threatening births were the two issues most often cited, for example: 'We know that it often is about life or death, and even if we are not doctors, we all know cases where the doctor has saved women from the certain death.'[38] For

33 Schiøtz, *Det offentlige helsevesen*, 187-95.

34 Stortingets forhandlinger (Parliamentary debate), 28th March 1933, 946.

35 Stortingets forhandlinger (Parliamentary debate), 28th March 1933, 951.

36 Cf. for instance local reports from the county of Søndre Bergenhus in Western Norway, *Søndre Bergenhus amtstings forhandlinger i aaret 1912*, A/S John Griegs boktrykkeri, Bergen, 631-32; *Søndre Bergenhus amtstings forhandlinger i aaret 1913*, A/S John Griegs boktrykkeri, Bergen, 286.

37 Stortingets forhandlinger (Parliamentary debate), 28th March1933, 946.

38 Stortingets forhandlinger (Parliamentary debate), 28th March 1933, 952.

that reason, the symbolic importance of the 'the doctor' in local communities was compared to 'the school' or access to stores; and the doctor was said to be the most important factor for where a liveable life was possible.[39] These services served as a mark of inclusion into 'modern' society, giving access to the common goods that were about to be regarded as necessities and, in regard of education and medical assistance, a public duty to provide.

These arguments say a great deal about changing perceptions of the quality and desirability of 'scientific medicine' and the services of medical practitioners among the rural populations – though only a generation earlier many had insisted that they had no need of doctors.[40] Such appreciation of medical practitioners and institutions was also expressed in the huge support received by voluntary associations working with health issues. In the first decades of the century, tens of thousands of members, largely women, rallied to civil associations such as *Norske Kvinners Sanitetsforening* (Norwegian Womens Public Health Association, established in 1896), *Den norske Nationalforening mot tuberkulosen* (The Norwegian National Association against Tuberculosis, established in 1910) and the Norwegian Red Cross, which picked up work on health issues after 1918. These associations mobilised in both urban and rural areas, in every part of the country: in 1923 the three organisations had approximately 193,000 members, rapidly increasing to 357,000 in 1936. They were highly active in the establishment and running of health institutions; they educated and employed local nurses and they conducted huge public enlightenment campaigns on health issues, as a rule in close cooperation with doctors and the state medical administration.[41]

Despite the protests, the numbers of MosH and medical districts were reduced in the period, as part of the annual parliamentary debate over the national budget, particularly where vacancies made possible the abolition of positions, mergers of medical districts, and reductions in salaries. Although the cutbacks in positions were not huge, from 393 in 1923 to 347 by 1934, the battles fought here reveal the importance attached to such posts. Interestingly, in some cases, the MosH themselves opted for abolition of positions and a merger of medical districts against the inclinations of local authorities.[42] This was partly because the communications revolution really had changed the situation and because in

---

39 Stortingets forhandlinger (Parliamentary debate), 29th March 1933, 970.

40 Andresen, A. and Ryymin, T. 'Towards Equality? Rural Health and Health Acts in Norway, 1860-1912', in Barona, J.L. and Cherry, S. (eds.) *Health and Medicine in Rural Europe (1850-1945)*. Valencia, PUV, Seminari d'Estudis Sobre la Ciència, 2005, 112-13, 125.

41 Schiøtz, *Det offentlige helsevesen*, 237-238.

42 Cf. St.prp. nr. 1, 1930, 2; 4; 68.

medical districts over a certain size the MoH was allowed to have some extra income in private practice, which encouraged interest in larger districts.

The economic crisis also affected the health institutions, whose proliferation had placed considerable financial strain on public funding and local health insurance societies. For instance, the expenses of the health insurance societies on hospital care had grown almost fivefold between 1916 and 1926, increasing the amount spent on hospital care from 9.7 per cent to 17.6 per cent of the insurance societies' total spending.[43] This growth reflected mainly the great number of new hospitals during the period. Restrictions on access to free hospital services were discussed but dismissed in 1928, as this, alongside access to doctors, was seen as the most important and effective part of the health insurance systems' services.[44] The main concession in reducing hospital care costs was that the reimbursement system was orientated around the public hospitals, with patient costs in private institutions tied to their public hospital equivalents.

However, the combination of economic crisis and changing perceptions of the medical adequacy of widely dispersed and small institutions during the 1920s and early 1930s, led to a new problematisation of such institutions and, indeed, of the whole hospital structure in Norway. The strained economy resulting from the numerous existing small institutions, planned, built and administered by medical doctors and local committees not necessarily versed in the art of rational architecture, was pointed out in the depths of depression in 1931-1932 by architect C. Thune-Larsen, according to whom cheaper and 'better' hospitals could only be achieved if experts were consulted.[45] Similar concerns were expressed by Professor Johan Holst, who argued for a planned division of labour between different types of hospitals. According to Holst, the increasingly specialised character of medicine necessitated a reform leading to a few big central hospitals, where the medical specialities were present, and a number of local hospitals where uncomplicated cases – such as 'purely surgical cases' – could be treated. A reform based on such a division of labour would attain the greatest possible medical efficiency for the lowest possible cost, stated Holst at the 25th annual meeting of the Norwegian Medical Association in 1934.[46]

---

43 Or in per capita terms, from 2,34 NOK to 11,04 NOK per insured member. Ot.prp. nr. 46 (1928) *Om å utferdige en lov om endringer i lov om sykeforsikring av 6. august 1915 med tilleggslover*. Appendix 1: *Innstilling fra Den departementale sykeforsikringskomité av 1927*, 40.

44 Ot.prp. nr. 46 (1928), 17; Ot.prp. nr. 46 (1928), Appendix 1, 42.

45 Thune-Larsen. C. 'Hvad der kan gjøres for økonomisering av våre sykehus's opførelse og drift', *Tidsskrift for Den norske lægeforening*, 51 (1931): 890-893; 'Økonomisk modernisering og utvidelse av sykehus', *Tidsskrift for Den norske lægeforening*, 52 (1932): 119-122.

46 Holst, J. 'Om organisasjonen av vårt offentlige sykehusvesen', *Tidsskrift for Den norske lægeforening*, 55 (1935): 302-311.

The Ministry of Social Affairs instigated in October 1934 a general survey of the existing medical institutions, which highlighted demands for such a centrally planned new hospital system.[47] The prevalence of small health institutions and lack of central direction in their establishment was branded as irrational by representatives of the state medical establishment. A replacement system would concentrate resources in well-equipped central hospitals able to deal with every kinds of sickness, with smaller hospitals 'equipped only for the most prevalent and usually occurring sicknesses' and located along communication lines – in accordance with Holst's argument.[48] The latter would serve as many patients as possible but were not equipped on par with the central hospitals.[49] So while small, locally initiated health institutions had previously been deemed adequate, indeed desirable, the new medical ideals emphasised the necessity of centralising resources to specialised institutions equipped with the state of the art medical technology and led by highly educated, medical specialists.[50]

Though such ideas were not particularly welcomed by medical practitioners affiliated with the smaller, older institutions, nor by local politicians, this was in fact how the hospital sector was to be remodelled after World War Two.[51] Nevertheless, in the most peripheral rural districts the cottage hospital was still deemed a necessity after the war, since otherwise the population would be left without hospital services.

Concluding remarks

Thus, the basis of the Norwegian health care system underwent a change from the beginning of the twentieth century to the early 1930s. Through the different acts passed between 1900 and 1912, the state had established a two-sided system of health care. First, local entrepreneurs, rural and urban, public and private alike, were encouraged to promote small, simple medical institutions in order to deal with the most pressing medical problems of that time. Through the 1900 TB and 1909 Sickness Insurance Acts, the state defined the economic supportive mechanisms that contributed to the viability of such local agencies, without central planning or direction. The institutions that developed over the following decades were established on local terms. Second, the state provided rural communities with a growing number of medical officers through the 1912 Pub-

47 Martinsen, *Omsorg, sykepleie og medisin*, 214-215.

48 Bu, *Sykehusene*, 1.

49 Bu, *Sykehusene*, 1-2.

50 A similar process was revealed in the wartime Hospital Surveys that informed planning of the British NHS. See Powell, M. 'Hospital Provision before the N.H.S.: A Geographic Study of the 1945 Hospital Surveys', in *Social History of Medicine*, 5, (3) (1992), 483-504.

51 Hansen, 'Sykehusstruktur', 40-44.

lic Medical Services Act. These state doctors were not only crucial for the proper scientific conduct of the many local health institutions, but were also in increasing demand by the rural population.

However, due to this system's very success, the resulting economic strain on public and private purses, (e.g. the sickness insurance societies), and rising expectations concerning medical facilities, meant that the underlying logic concerning the primacy of local agency became contested. The system of equalisation and enhancement of health care via sickness insurance and local hospital building was branded as a problem by the central medical authorities during the 1920s and early 1930s. In 1934, attempts were made to increase the level of state direction within the health care system; with plans for a new, centralised hospital structure drafted and the 1912 Act modified to allow greater central direction of where state medical officers served.

The establishment of medical institutions could perhaps be characterised as a transferral of the logic of individual self-help in the field of social welfare to a community level: local agency by voluntary associations and municipal authorities to provide health services through medical institutions was encouraged through financial mechanisms built into the TB and Health insurance acts. This activity was in part to be guided by the medical officers of health and other state-authorised health officials, but by and large decisions about what kind of institutions to build or their location were local ones. In the early 1930s, however, centrally defined expert knowledge on these matters and on where doctors were most needed had gained ground over local agency – and partly, this happened in the name of equality.

Equality and universalism had been central in the establishment of the health care system in the first decade of the century. At that time universalism was the result of an intervention by rural interests in the formation of the health care acts. For instance the Health Insurance Act gradually came to encompass large segments of rural population in order to counteract a transferral of resources from the countryside to deal with the problems of the urban working class. Furthermore, it was rural interests that in 1912 had determined that the country should be divided into such a large number of medical districts. This form of universalism reflected rural economic and political strength, but the universalism of the post-1945 health care system was now largely motivated by conceived weaknesses of the countryside. Rural economic and political strength had greatly diminished during the economic crisis and, despite the continuing importance of MosH and the small rural medical institutions, it was now the large and specialised hospitals that were regarded as essential to advanced medical effort and achieving the best forms of health care.

GENERAL HOSPITAL SERVICES FOR RURAL AND PERIPHERAL AREAS OF NORWAY 1920-1950

Tore Grønlie

To discuss general hospital development and organisation in Norway with the focus upon services for the rural or peripheral population is no straightforward undertaking. No comprehensive study of the hospitals for this period exists, whether nationwide or on a county or regional (*landsdel*) basis.[1] Only a few specialised studies deal with elements of the hospital system, if that word is appropriate here.[2] Individual hospital studies do exist, but few are systematised or placed within the perspective of national hospital development.[3] This paper thus represents a first outline of the urban-rural distribution of general hospital services in Norway in the decades from 1920 to 1950 and it highlights some problems for further research. In doing so, it omits the mental hospitals and tuberculosis institutions that, in fact, comprised the bulk of institutions in rural areas.[4]

---

1 The five natural geographical regions being south, west, east, north and 'mid'- Norway. A comprehensive study of the public health system does exist, it is more concerned, however, with public health policy, than with institutions, Schiøtz, A. *Det offentlige helsevesen i Norge 1603-2003. Folkets helse - landets styrke 1850-2003*, Oslo, Universitetsforlaget, 2003.

2 It could very well be argued that a national system of hospital services did not exist before regionalization and state take over of hospitals in 2002.

3 For example Elster, T. *Rikets hospital : historien om et lite samfunn i den store verden*, Oslo, Aschehoug, 1990; Janssen, C. W. *Haukeland sykehus : en medisinsk hjørnesten siden 1912* [utgitt i samarbeid med Informasjonsavdelingen, Haukeland sykehus], Bergen, Eide, 2001; Reiersen, *E. L. Sykehuset Sanitetsforeningen Lokalsamfunnet Orkdal Sanitetsforenings Sjukehus 1909-1984*, Orkanger, Orkdal sanitetsforening, 1985; Jacobsen, T. *Fra sneppert til skalpell. Sykehushistorie i Rana gjennom hundre år*, Mo i Rana, Rana sykehus, 2001.

4 Classifications are difficult, as many institutions were combined hospitals for general cases and tuberculosis. Small hospitals also often started out as a tuberculosis institution, was developed into a combined hospital for tuberculosis and general diseases and ended up as a general hospital. We have concentrated on institutions catering only or mainly for general cases. The source material used in this article obviously also focuses services in general hospitals of 'some size' and with a minimum of specialization. This goes a long way towards explaining any discrepancies between this article and that by Andresen and Ryymin (see above), which is more concerned with the full magnitude of rural health institutions and services.

The focus is upon how the general hospital needs of rural or peripheral populations were actually met, relative to those of urban dwellers. Definitions of urban, rural or peripheral populations are of major importance in any study and findings will depend greatly upon definitions. With limits upon source materials and available space, the focus here will be mainly on the question of differences between counties, and the relationships between clearly urban and non-urban areas within a particular county. Discussion centres upon three important features: access to hospitals, expenses and payments for hospital treatment, and hospital quality. The emphasis will be on access, as the essential element of hospital services, and since more research exists concerning this feature than the other two.

Map 1. Norway 1934: Distances, populations and hospital beds per 1000 inhabitants by counties

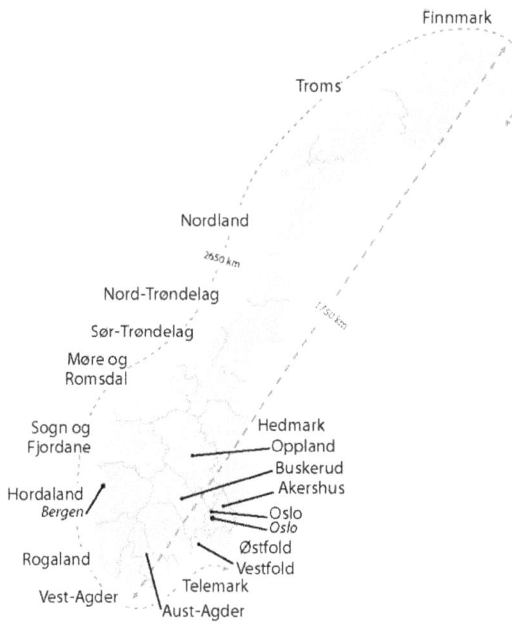

Area: 325 000 km2. Population: 11 per km2. Hospital beds per 1000 inhabitants: County spread 2-4, Oslo 9, Bergen 6. Source: Bu 1941.

Access

How far is it possible to give a reasonably precise picture of access to hospitals for rural or peripheral populations? National statistics on aggregate levels give few clues. A comparison between the country's 20 counties in the mid 1930s reveals no great or systematic differences in the distribution of hospital beds. Oslo and Bergen, the two main cities and both counties in their own right, had hospital bed ratios of nine and six per 1,000 inhabitants respectively, although – as we shall see – these serviced much larger populations than their own. Most other counties offered between two and four hospital beds per 1,000 and there were no systematic differences between more densely or sparsely populated counties.[5]

Study of the hospitals' localities, whether in rural or small town areas or in cities, in isolation from other important factors, does not take us much further. General hospitals of any size are almost by nature an urban phenomenon. Most are situated in population centres and those in genuinely rural locations are exceptional, contrary to the usual experience with mental hospitals and institutions for the treatment of tuberculosis. Ease of access for the majority of patients and their families within a reasonably sized catchment area meant that even hospitals servicing mainly rural or peripheral populations were usually established in population centres or in the suburban areas. This general tendency is probably of even greater importance in a country as sparsely populated and geographically subdivided as Norway. Access thus involves not simply the geographical localisation of hospitals in predominantly rural or small town settings and their intended patient clientele, but also the extent and conditions under which rural populations might also be serviced by city hospitals established mainly for their own populations.

In a country as geographically widespread, diverse and sub-divided as Norway, hospital access might have been *the* main problem for the rural or peripheral areas, yet the first general survey of hospital services from 1934 leaves a rather different impression. The state county governors (*fylkesmenn*), leading officials of local authorities, county medical officers (*fylkeslegene*) and state medical officers of health (*distriktslegene*) of almost all 20 counties generally agreed that access to hospitals in their respective counties was satisfactory or good, albeit first and foremost for more common illnesses and surgery. The few counties where access was reported as unsatisfactory were balanced by those with very good conditions and there were few systematic differences between sparcely and more densely populated counties. In Hordaland, a highly diverse county with a relatively big, scattered, rural population, the county medical officer ascertained that 'nobody suffered ('ikke si at noen lider nød') or was exposed to risk.'[6] The state county governor of Hedmark, another geographically widespread county, reported that it was 'very well equipped' ('meget godt utstyrt') with hospital beds.[7] Other statements reveal that local authority and medical officials generally attributed satisfactory or good access to the hospital expansion of recent decades; a very much decentralised pattern of hospital

5 Bu, S. *Sykehusene i Norge*, Oslo, Chr. Gundersens boktrykkeri, 1941, Table 2, Hospital beds by county 1934.

6 Bu, *Sykehusene*, 58-105, citation, 84.

7 Bu, *Sykehusene*, 64.

establishment; and hospital admission policies that were generally solidaristic in principle.[8]

What influenced these developments? Norway had no general hospital law before 1969 and until then no single authority was assigned the responsibility for the building and running of general hospitals.[9] This contrasted with neighbouring Sweden, so often misleadingly depicted as representing a Scandinavian model, where responsibility for hospitals was placed with the counties as early as 1864 and remains so.[10] It also differed from Britain, where general hospitals were largely entrusted to the voluntary sector and responsibility for the poor-law hospitals rested with local authorities in a dual system until the late 1920s, eventually replaced by the unitary state National Health Service from 1948.[11] Arrangements in Norway, seen by some as 'almost anarchic', might best be characterised as a collaborative effort, a process of 'chipping in', pooling whatever resources could be found and activated, both locally and nationwide.[12] This in turn, reflected a 'Norwegian system', under which collective services were often funded from a variety of sources during the nineteenth century.[13] Different combinations of public and private interests and authorities could be found behind local hospital initiatives; local or county authorities, private humanitarian or religious organisations, or ad hoc interest groups and even companies. With regard to its general hospitals, the early Norwegian welfare state owed little to the state

8 Bu, *Sykehusene*, 58-105. Schiøtz states that more than 100 'mixed' ('blandede') hospitals, out of may be around 250 in total, were built in the 1920s and 1930s. Schiøtz, *Det offentlige helsevesen*, 320. Note that this suggests another important element of the success story, as also outlined by Andresen and Ryymin above.

9 E.g. Martinsen, K. 'Helsepolitiske problemer og helsepolitisk tenkning bak sykehusloven av 1969', *Historisk tidsskrift* 3-1987; Grønlie, T. 'Norwegian General Hospitals, 1970–2002: County Ownership—An Interlude between Welfare Localism and State Direction', *Medical History*, 2006; 50(2): 189-208.

10 Haave, P. 'The Hospital Sector: a Four-Country Comparison of Organisational and Political Development', in Christiansen, N. F.; Petersen, K.; Edling, N.; Haave, P. (eds.) *The Nordic Model of welfare. A Historic Reappraisal*, Copenhagen, Museum Tusculanum Press, 2006, 218-20; Angell, S.I. 'Two variants of decentralized health care: Norway and Sweden in comparison', Bergen, Stein Rokkan Centre, 2009. Submitted for publication in Medical History.

11 Eg. Mohan, J. *Planning, Markets and Hospitals*, London and New York, 2002; Webster, C. *The National Health Service. A Political History*. 2nd Edition, Oxford, 2002; Grønlie, T. 'Hospital Sector Structure and Organization in Britain and Norway – Contributions Towards a Comparative Study', in Andresen, A.; Elvbakken, K.T, and Grønlie, T. (eds.) *Politics of Prevention, Health Propaganda, and the Organisation of Hospitals*, Conference Proceedings. Rokkan Report 10, Bergen, Stein Rokkan Centre, 2005.

12 Grønlie, T. 'Norwegian General Hospitals', 193, quoting Hansen, F. H. (ed). *SAMDATA. Sykehus Rapport. Sykehusstruktur i endring. De lange linjene og utviklingen siste tiår*. Trondheim, SINTEF Unimed NIS SAMDATA/Kommuneforlaget, 2001, 38.

13 E.g. Seip, J. A. *Tanke og handling i norsk politikk*, Oslo, Gyldendal, 1968, 22-71. 1968.

itself.[14] The state owned and ran the National hospital (*Rikshospitalet*) in the capital city of Oslo, a few military hospitals and specialist institutions, notably maternity clinics in Oslo and Bergen, tuberculosis sanatoria and mental hospitals. It also contributed to national health insurance, implemented in 1911 (see below) and made sporadic direct hospital investment. Historically, and arguably until the 1970s, there were no provisions or mechanisms to secure any even or otherwise systematic nationwide distribution of hospitals.

In 1930 only eight per cent of general hospital beds were in state institutions, with 11 per cent more in hospitals owned by the counties. By comparison 51 per cent of hospital beds were in institutions owned by local authorities, in addition to nine per cent in those jointly owned by local and county authorities and 21 per cent in private ownership, most often religious or humanitarian organisations.[15] If local authorities predominated as hospital builders and owners, the principal actors here were the cities and the larger towns. The expression 'local authority welfare' or 'welfare municipality' (*velferdskommunen*) commonly denotes their pioneering effort long before the state had any dominant role in welfare production and distribution.[16] Although primary health services reflected significant state intervention, hospital building and administration remained an important and integral part of local authority welfare.[17] Extensive hospital expansion followed late nineteenth-century urbanisation, in which the bigger cities, notably Oslo, Bergen and Trondheim, were prominent, their 'municipal socialism' reflecting the leading role of leftist parties.[18] However, mid-sized cities and towns also followed suit after World War One and throughout the 1920s.[19]

Hospital investment was greatly inspired and eased by the contributions to amortisation and interest payment by national health insurance.[20] But the driving force was welfare localism, under which locally defined needs were largely met by local efforts.[21] The involvement of cities and towns in hospitals was not in

---

14 Grønlie, 'Norwegian General Hospitals'; Hansen, *SAMDATA. Sykehus Rapport.*

15 National statistics, NOS IX.2, after Grønlie, 'Norwegian General Hospitals', 193.

16 Eg. Grønlie, T. 'Velferdskommune og utjevningsstat', in Næss, H. E.; Hovland, E.; Danielsen, R.; Grønlie, T. and Baldersheim, H. *Folkestyre i by og bygd*, Oslo, Bergen, Stavanger, Tromsø, Universitetsforlaget 1987; Grønlie, T. 'Velferdskommunen', in Nagel, A. H. (ed.) *Velferdskommunen. Kommunenes rolle i utviklingen av velferdsstaten*, Bergen, Alma Mater, 1991; Grønlie, T. 'Fra velferdskommune til velferdsstat – hundre års velferdsvekst fra lokalisme til statsdominans', *Historisk tidsskrift* bd. 83, 4, 2004, 633-649.

17 Grønlie, 'Norwegian General Hospitals'.

18 Danielsen, R. 'Kommunaliseringsprosessen i norske byer 1880-1920', in Nagel (ed.) *Velferdskommunen*. Flo, Y. *Staten og sjølvstyret*. Dr. art. avhandling, Universitetet i Bergen, 2004.

19 E.g. Schiøtz, *Det offentlige helsevesen*, 320-24.

20 Haave, 'The Hospital Sector', 222-23.

21 Schiøtz, *Det offentlige helsevesen*, 320-24, Grønlie, 'Norwegian General Hospitals', 192.

response to any national decree, plan or political drive, but reflected local appreciation of need and utilisation of local taxation as a resource, even though urban authorities had neither jurisdiction nor responsibilities beyond their own boundaries. There was no state coordination.

In principle, then, each local authority was left on its own. There were major economic and cultural differences between most of the 750 or so local authorities (*kommuner*) that were rural and peripheral, with populations of a few thousands or less, compared with larger towns or cities. Only a minority of smaller local authorities could act as independent welfare authorities but some cooperated with neighbouring communities or public or private agencies to build small cottage hospitals (*sykestuer* or *sykehjem*), an important facility, when communication with urban centres were especially difficult. [22] By 1934-35 there were between 40 and 50 such institutions, typically of less than 20 beds, under varying forms of ownership and usually located in peripheral areas affected by difficult communications.[23] In some cases groups of local authorities also worked together to finance or contribute towards the building of a larger common hospital.

Where the great mass of smaller local authorities could not act as hospital providers independently or severally, the county authority could take on this role. From the introduction of local self-government in 1837 local authorities were also members of the county authority, which was primarily an institution of support for rural communities. As already seen, county authorities in the 1930s figured among the bigger hospital builders and owners and only two, Akershus and Hordaland, lacked a county hospital.[24] Nevertheless, the county role in hospital provision was disproportionately low, considering the rural-urban distribution of the population in Norway. Why was this? With no obligation to build hospitals before 1969, the will to engage in costly welfare institutions was generally much less evident at the county level than in cities and towns, as were the resources available for such ventures. The county authority, composed of the mayors of the member communities, depended on taxes levied indirectly on the local communities and tended to concentrate on basic or affordable services, with an eye to keeping down costs and the tax burden on member constituencies. In geographically diverse counties there were conflicting interests over the location of county hospitals since larger and more well-to-do communities – often relatively densely populated areas bordering on a hospital town or city – had little interest in funding services or care focused upon the less fortunate of the periphery.[25] Thus appeals to the merits of welfare localism stood less chance of success in the county assembly than in the cities and towns.

---

22 Grønlie, T. 'Velferdskommune og utjevningsstat'
23 Bu, *Sykehusene*, table 1, 22-35.
24 Bu, *Sykehusene*, 59, 84.
25 Grønlie, 'Norwegian General Hospitals', 194.

Yet hospital access for rural and peripheral populations was not restricted to the extent indicated by the municipal-county hospital balance. To understand why, we need to consider the different actors and functions of the hospital system. Although urban local authorities were predominant in hospital building, their own requirements did not exclude rural populations in their surrounding areas. In fact patients from such areas were regularly treated by urban local authority hospitals and enjoyed much the same rights as the municipalities' own inhabitants. In the county of Østfold, for example, 25-60 per cent of patients in town hospitals came from rural areas, especially so from neighbouring districts and in Buskerud some 60 per cent of the patients in town institutions were rural dwellers.[26] Local authorities in the vicinity of cities and towns sometimes participated in the planning and financing of urban hospitals which from the outset were meant to service the greater area. To a lesser extent such hospitals also accommodated patients from beyond a county, if it were easier and cheaper for these to travel across county borders than inside their own county. Thus patients from coastal areas in the south-western Hordaland usually sought hospital treatment in the town of Haugesund, in neighbouring Rogaland county, because of difficult communications with Bergen, their 'own' hospital city. Similarly, one-half of the county population of Sogn og Fjordane was said to have easier southward access to Bergen, than to the 'hospital town' of Florø, in the far western part of their own county.[27]

The Haukeland Sykehus was Bergen's local authority hospital and the largest hospital outside of Oslo. During the mid-1930s and early 1950s around 25 per cent of its patients came from outside the city, from the county of Hordaland, covering the coast, fjord and inland area around and east of Bergen, from Sogn and Fjordane to the north or other counties of West Norway.[28] Most of Hordaland was within acceptable travelling distance from Bergen, and its population relied heavily on the neighbouring 'hospital city' as there was no county hospital and less than one hospital bed per 1,000 persons.[29] Though Hordaland for years had plans for a county hospital, and even acquired a building site in Bergen, these never came to fruition.[30] These and other examples suggest that equal access for rural populations to urban local authority hospitals was more the rule than the exception.

---

26 Bu, *Sykehusene*, 62.

27 Bu, *Sykehusene*, 87.

28 Bu, *Sykehusene*, 82; Grønlie, T. 'Bergen bys historie 1945-1972', in: Grønlie, T. and Fossen, A.B. *Bergen bys historie IV. Byen sprenger grensene 1920-1972.* Universitetsforlaget, Oslo, 1985, 793.

29 Bu, *Sykehusene*, table 2, 56, p. 84.

30 Bu, *Sykehusene*, 84-85.

Almost one-quarter of general hospital beds in 1934 were provided by non-public organisations, usually humanitarian or religious in outlook but often acting in different combinations with public authorities and funded partly from public and national health insurance sources. Historically the Norwegian 'welfare triangle' featured tripartite partnership between local authorities, organisations and the state.[31] How did this affect the country's rural and peripheral populations? Around 70 per cent of private hospital beds were owned by secular non-profit, humanitarian organisations, like the Red Cross or the Women's Sanitary Organization (*Norske Kvinners Sanitetsforening*) and there was no distinct urban-rural pattern in their distribution of hospitals. Hospital building was initiated and carried through by local branches to fill local needs, with both large and small institutions in city, small town and rural environments, though in quite a few cases they filled important peripheral needs.[32] The group of secular hospital owners also included private mining or prime metal companies, often under obligation by state concessionary requirements to build hospitals for their workers. Their hospitals were usually located in small 'company towns' in the periphery, such as Sauda on the west coast.

Religious organisations provided just below 30 per cent of the private general hospital beds.[33] The hospital engagement of religious organisations and denominations was first and foremost a city phenomenon. In 1934, for example, all 18 Catholic hospitals were urban, but again these offered care to non-urban patients. The urban-rural ratio of Norway's private religious hospital patients is unknown but, discussing the religious organisations in 1934-35, the county medical officer of Hordaland (fylkeslegen) felt that 'The private clinics in Bergen are always ready to receive everybody who needs hospital care from the county of Hordaland'.[34] Indeed from 1930 to 1936, between 65 and almost 90 per cent of the capacity in private hospitals in Bergen was utilised by out-of-city occupants.[35] Perhaps this was because the public hospital in Bergen was overburdened and lacked resources to increase services during the depression of the 1930s, whereas the private hospitals expanded considerably. Arguably then,

---

31 Seip, A.L.'Velferdskommunen og velferdstrekanten – et tilbakeblikk', in Nagel (ed.) *Velferdskommunen.*

32 Eg. Reiersen, *Sykehuset Sanitetsforeningen Lokalsamfunnet*; Jacobsen, *Fra sneppert til skalpell*; Hamran , T. 'Kvinneforeningene, institusjonsbyggingen og den nasjonale velferdspolitikken. Nord-Norge før 1940'. *Historisk Tidsskrift* vol. 86, 3, 2007, 411-430.

33 Bu, *Sykehusene*, 18, table 8, 56. Figures here cover all hospitals, both general, psychiatric and hospitals for other special needs. Catholic orders provided roughly 60 % and the protestant ones 40%.

34 Bu, *Sykehusene*, 84.

35 Measured by 'days in bed'. Fossen, A.B. 'Tiden 1920-1945', in Fossen and Grønlie, *Bergen bys historie*, 302.

Bergen's private hospitals effectively specialised in meeting the acute medical needs of Hordaland's rural population.

Map 2. Problematic access to hospitals due to difficult communications – 1934 (Unit: Medical districts)

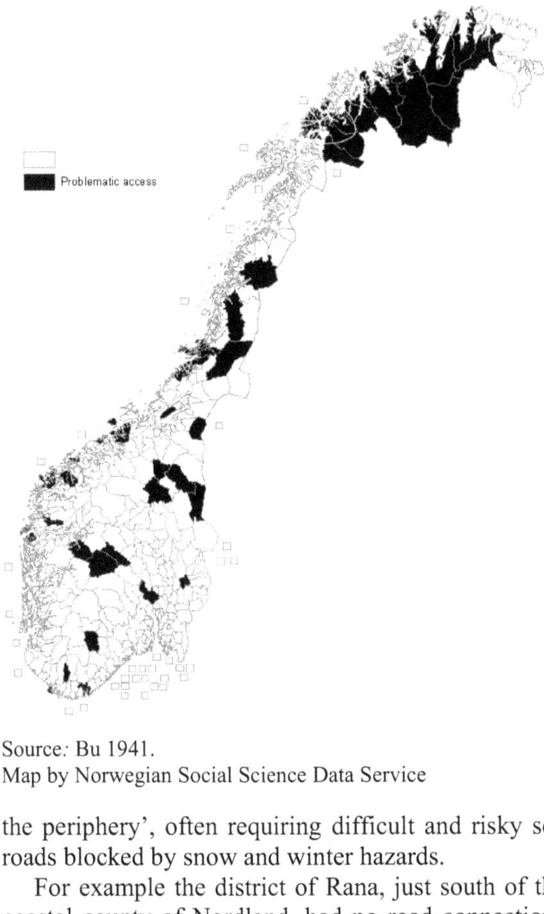

Source: Bu 1941.
Map by Norwegian Social Science Data Service

A reasonable conclusion so far is that satisfaction with hospital access was widespread and general – in most counties. Yet some rural populations did face communications problems, with unsatisfactory, long, complicated or even dangerous journeys to county hospital towns. Particularly affected were the northern counties of Finnmark and Nordland; Nord-Trøndelag in Mid-Norway; Møre and Romsdal and Sogn og Fjordane in the west, and some peripheral inland areas of Eastern Norway.[36] These more remote areas, generally singled out by their respective district medical officials, could possibly be called 'the periphery of the periphery', often requiring difficult and risky sea transportation, or having roads blocked by snow and winter hazards.

For example the district of Rana, just south of the Arctic Circle in the long coastal county of Nordland, had no road connections to the county hospital in the coastal small town of Sandnessjøen, and no winter connections with the county hospital in Bodø, almost 250 km to the north. The fjord steamer took patients on the 70-80 km long Ranafjord, along what was locally called the appendicitis route (*blindtarmruta*).[37] This spurred the local branch of the

36 Bu, *Sykehusene*, 58-105.
37 Jacobsen, *Fra sneppert til skalpell*, 38-46.

Women's Sanitary Organisation to great voluntary efforts to build a hospital, having already realised their ambition of building a local tuberculosis institution. The hospital opened in 1942 with 20 beds, expanding to 50 in the early 1950s and around 100 a decade later. Prime responsibility for its management gradually passed over to public authorities, however, and a new hospital under county direction was erected in the mid 1960s.[38] Even then, patients requiring specialised or complex acute services and complicated births cases were transported by ambulance to Namsos, 350 km to the south, often under bad wintery road conditions. Hospital treatment under these circumstances would obviously be sought only in the most serious and acute cases, although aggregate data does not allow precise measurement of the magnitude of these problems.

Costs and payments

It is not yet possible to provide a comprehensive and reasonably precise description of how hospital costs were financed, neither by the providers nor patients. However a combination of national figures and local studies offers some indications and research pointers. From 1911 a system of national health insurance, organised through local health insurance societies (*kretssykekasser*), provided both cash and medical benefits, including hospital services, for the insured and their family members.[39] Some 60 per cent of insurance costs were paid by the insured person, with a 20 per cent state contribution and a further ten per cent each coming from the local authority and the employer.[40] The most important membership criteria from the outset was employment, as self-employed persons in agriculture, fisheries, handicrafts and other groups, all common occupations in rural areas, were excluded. Gradually, though, membership was expanded, from over 30 per cent of the working population in 1912, to roughly 65 per cent in 1938, 70-75 per cent in 1948, and 90 per cent by 1956, when health insurance became obligatory.[41]

In principle, health insurance covered the full costs of hospital care in all hospitals, irrespective of ownership. Hospitals were refunded their costs on the

---

38 Jacobsen, *Fra sneppert til skalpell*, 47-75. Cf. Reiersen, *Sykehuset Sanitetsforeningen Lokalsamfunnet*.

39 Bjørnson, Ø. and Haavet, I. E. *Langsomt ble landet et velferdssamfunn. Trygdens historie 1894-1994*, Ad Notam/Gyldendal, Oslo, 1994, 55-79; Haave, 'The Hospital Sector', 220-23.

40 Bjørnson and Haavet, *Langsomt ble landet*, 69.

41 Bjørnson and Haavet, *Langsomt ble landet*, 72-79, Seip, A.L. *Veiene til velferdsstaten. Norsk sosialpolitikk 1920-75*, Oslo, Gyldendal, 1994, 198-206. Fishermen became members in 1935 and seamen in foreign waters in 1940, self-employed farmers, smallholders and craftsmen not until 1956. Cash benefits for the self-employed were made obligatory only in 1970.

basis of rates initially meant to cover care on a day-to day basis (*kurpenger, liggedøgnsrefusjon*). Everywhere charges for out-of-town patients from the county in which the host town or city was situated appear to have been the same as for urban dwellers. For out-of-county patients, however, it was a relatively common practice nationwide to charge somewhat more.[42] Non-members had to cover their own expenses, with poorer patients seeking social support from their respective local authorities' health or poor relief budgets. Payments to public institutions were usually based upon set day-to-day rates collected for members. Patients in private hospitals themselves had to cover the difference between their usually higher day rates and those refunded by health insurance. Non-members either paid in full out of their own purse or sought social benefits.[43] We do not know the extent to which charges were really collected by the humanitarian non-profit hospitals from patients with little or no ability to pay.

Yet it seems that rural or peripheral populations were more heavily burdened than urban ones, for a number of reasons. First, for several decades rural dwellers, more likely to be self-employed or in occupations not covered by health insurance, fell outside the scheme and so needed to raise the money themselves or ask for public support, which no doubt made them less likely to seek hospital services. This is clearly demonstrated by an example from the county of Nordland. This county had a large fishermen population and its medical officer stated in 1939 that assessments made five years earlier, that hospital capacity and access were satisfactory, were already outdated. In 1935 fishermen had been included in the health insurance scheme, which had changed the situation 'totally' since access was now problematic and hospitals were in need of expansion.[44] Apparently the extension of health insurance had greatly enhanced demand for hospital treatment.

Second, if it is generally true that rural inhabitants were over-represented at private hospitals, they might incur higher costs than town-dwellers, either as insured members required to pay higher day rates, or as non-members presented with full charges. The county medical officer and the officers of the health insurance boards in Hordaland, for example, generally complained about the high day rates at Bergen hospitals and charges for extra services on top of the doctors' pay.[45] Indeed these complaints were important factors behind the county's aborted plan to establish its own hospital.[46] Third, it is likely that non-members

42 Bu, *Sykehusene*, table 3, 6. 'Kurpenger pr. døgn'.

43 We do not know much of the actual, probably highly different, practises nationwide. Here we lean on knowledge of conditions in Bergen, cf. Fossen, 'Bergen bys historie1920-1945', 296-303.

44 Bu, *Sykehusene*, 100, cf. Bjørnson and Haavet, *Langsomt ble landet*, 72.

45 Bu, *Sykehusene*, 84.

46 Bu, *Sykehusene*, 84.

of the health insurance scheme in cities and towns had easier access to public funds to meet hospital charges than those in less wealthy rural communities. Moreover, travelling costs represented a significant additional burden for people in rural and peripheral area.

In practice, however, day-to-day rates often did not nearly cover the real costs in hospitals, and this ironically may have actually favoured rural populations. In Bergen, for instance, health insurance in 1930-31 covered only about 63 per cent of real costs at the city hospital, and ten years later around 75 per cent. The result was that local authority hospitals ran up big deficits that had to be paid out of tax moneys.[47] We do not know much about how this problem was solved nationally but it is clear that, in Bergen at least, the city for a long time was a more than reasonable hospital owner, when considered from the urban-rural perspective. Because the city covered the hospital deficit itself, it effectively subsidised the patients from neighbouring or outlying rural or small town areas. It has been suggested that cities and towns viewed hospitals and other social and cultural institutions, not only as an obligation, but also as status symbols (*adelsmerke*) or privileges. Hospitals contributed to the making of a town or a city and towns lacking these kinds of institutions were of a lower order, a feature which probably spurred them to raise their status. At the same time, having a hospital implied an obligation to extend this form of care to people in surrounding rural areas and smaller towns. Thus the larger towns and cities contributed to the welfare of others 'out of their riches'.[48] As the head of the Bergen hospital administration put it in 1934-5;

> 'The local authority hospital in Bergen has for a long time functioned as central hospital for large parts of West Norway. The city has felt this to be a natural task, as the centre for big rural areas, whose needs for hospital accommodation could not without great difficulties be met in other places than here. ... For great parts of the county of Hordaland it seems natural that Bergen also in the future has to be the centre for hospital treatment. And there are no reasons to believe that the city will change its hospital policies, if not dictated by enforcing economic or other restraints.' [49]

Some 20 years later, as the second university in Norway was established in Bergen, the city was even more eager to develop its position as a leading hospital centre of West Norway. However, the days of subsidising the rural and peripheral areas were over: from 1952 Hordaland had to pay the deficits of the

---

47 Fossen, 'Bergen bys historie 1920-1945', 297-303; Grønlie, 'Bergen bys historie 1945-1972', 788-98.

48 Grønlie, 'Norwegian General Hospitals', 193-94.

49 Bu, *Sykehusene*, 83.

county's own patients, who in the mid-1960s comprised almost half of those in the Bergen city hospital.[50]

Quality

Hospital access, as we have seen, was not considered a great problem, except in the most remote areas, where communications with the urban centres were especially difficult. Hospital charges posed greater difficulty for rural populations, especially those excluded from health insurance, but what about the quality of services? No figures measuring quality of treatment exist. We will very briefly consider two indicators of quality; the degree of specialisation, and the possibility of transfer to hospitals of a higher order, when local hospitals had no recognised or specialist treatment to offer. In the late 1930s the degree of specialisation remained very low indeed. Even in 1946, Norway's health director, Karl Evang, was of the opinion that only two hospitals in all of Norway, the National Hospital and Ullevål Hospital (the municipal authority hospital), both in Oslo, qualified for the new status of central hospital (*sentralsykehus*), in that they employed specialists in all important sub-disciplines of hospital medicine. Moreover just one hospital, the Haukeland Sykehus, the upcoming university clinic in Bergen, was a candidate for such status.[51] There were then roughly 250 general hospitals of all sizes in Norway, but outside of Oslo these had only around 120 specialists.[52] Most of the latter were surgeons, 70 of whom worked in 62 hospitals or hospital departments, reflecting the strong position of surgery from the turn of the century. Moreover new or modernised hospitals were usually built primarily as clinics of surgery, and for two or three decades hospital treatment was identified by most people primarily with acute surgical work, often in accident cases.[53] Most counties, including the less urbanised, reported that the capacity for surgical treatment was good or satisfactory.[54] Yet there were surgeons

---

50 Grønlie, 'Bergen bys historie 1945-1972', 788-98.

51 Evang, K. 'Norsk sykehuspolitikk', *Liv og helse: norsk blad for riktig levesett*, No. 1946, 256-61.

52 Schiøtz, *Det offentlige helsevesen*, 320, Bu, *Sykehusene*, 18. This excludes around 150 institutions for mental illness and tuberculosis, and their relevant specialists. Statistics are problematic: the figure of 197 specialists (53 in tuberculosis and 24 in mental illness) in 1934 is for the counties outside Oslo. In Oslo's National and Ullevål hospitals, it is known only that there were specialists in all departments.

53 Hospitals with the sole speciality of surgery, but also caring for patients with other ills, were usually called 'mixed hospitals' (blandede sykehus). Schiøtz, *Det offentlige helsevesen*, 320. Schiøtz reports that more of 100 of these were built in the 1920s and 1930s. On the expansion of surgery, see Schiøtz, *Det offentlige helsevesen*, 320; Bu, *Sykehusene*, 97 (statement from the county medical officer of Nord-Trøndelag).

54 Bu, *Sykehusene*, 50-100. See also Bu's general statement: 'capacity at hospitals for surgery is satisfactory in most counties.' Bu, *Sykehusene*, 8.

only at big or mid-sized hospitals – one-quarter of the total – and rarely more than one in each institution. Two counties had only one hospital or department led by a surgeon, four counties had two, while the rest had between three and five.[55]

The situation was far less satisfactory in other specialities, and here the urban-peripheral dimension is very much visible. In all of Norway outside of Oslo there were only 16 specialists in (internal) medicine. Complaints over the lack of capacity for treatment in (internal) medicine came from more than half of the counties.[56] The problem was greatest in counties with no specialisation in medicine at all with eight counties, almost all in the coastal west, the north or the less-urbanised areas of the east in this category.[57] There were only 34 other specialists outside of Oslo, eleven of them in radiology.[58] With just five specialists in the whole country in gynaecology or obstetrics, eleven counties had neither special hospitals nor hospital departments for childbirth or gynaeco-

Map 3. Counties with no specialists in internal medicine (1934)

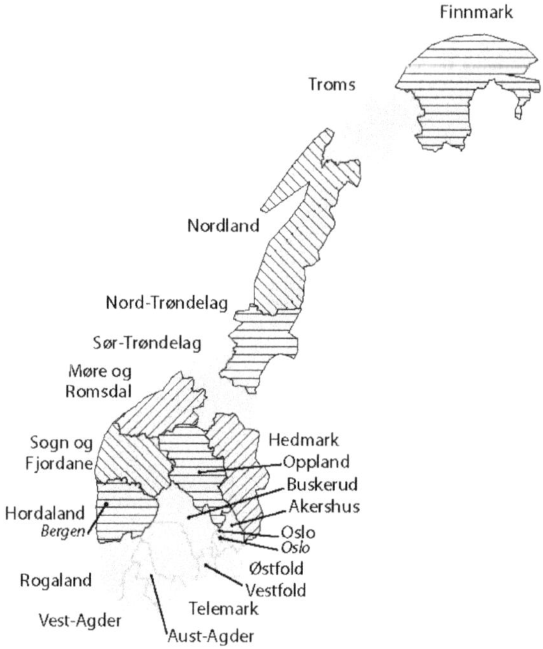

Source: Bu 1941.

55 Bu, *Sykehusene*, 7.

56 Bu, *Sykehusene*, 8-9, 50-100.

57 Hedmark, Oppland, Hordaland, Sogn og Fjordane, Møre og Romsdal, Nord-Trøndelag, Nordland og Finnmark. Bu, *Sykehusene*, 8-9.

58 Bu, *Sykehusene*, 20-21.'Mixed hospitals' in the range of 100-120 beds were usually upgraded to 'hospitals of three specialities' (tre-delte sykehus), surgery, medicine and radiology. Schiøtz, *Det norske helsevesen*, 320.

logical treatments, most of these in the same regions as those lacking specialists in (internal) medicine.[59] Meanwhile, specialists in orthopaedics, chil-dren's diseases, eye, ear, nose and throat and neurology were virtually non-existent.[60]

Given this situation, what were the possibilities of qualified treatment at a more advanced institution than the relevant local one? This is an under-researched area. There was no formal hierarchy of hospitals and no formal regionalisation above the local level.[61] In theory, the National Hospital in Oslo was open for all specialised treatments not finding solutions locally, but how this functioned in practice is unclear.[62] Reports for the mid-1930s from northern, western and southern Norway simply did not refer to the National Hospital as an alternative at all. We do not know why. Certainly its capacity was small and the possibilities of coming to Oslo from far-away counties were limited. A multi-day journey combining the coastal steamer and the railway was required for anyone from the far north, so it is likely that the National Hospital was first and foremost a specialist institution for patients from south-east Norway. Yet although it was mentioned frequently in reports by district medical officers from local peripheral areas of the south-eastern counties, relatively near to Oslo, this was always framed negatively, in terms of difficult or denied access and long waiting periods or lists.

Bergen's hospitals, notably the municipal Haukeland Sykehus, offered specialist treatment for most of western Norway. The 1934 survey suggested that the western counties were more satisfied with the Bergen solution, when compared with the eastern counties and the National Hospital. The county medical officer of Sogn og Fjordane, bordering on Bergen and Hordaland to the north, reported: 'Till this day it has never been difficult having patients needing *specialised treatment* admitted to hospitals in Bergen.'[63] Like his colleagues in Hordaland, he was more worried about costs for the county and the patients, than for access. Of a medical hierarchy in southern Norway, mid-Norway and Northern Norway, we know very little, but hospitals in Kristiansand (south), Stavanger (south-west), Trondheim (mid-Norway), and Tromsø (north Norway) probably had some specialised functions for areas outside their normal circumference, though not to be equated with Oslo – or Bergen.

---

59 Bu, *Sykehusene*, 15.

60 Bu, *Sykehusene*, 19-20.

61 A formalized regionalized system was established – on paper – only in the mid-1970s. Only after a state take-over of all hospitals in 2002 was regionalization put into effect through a regional decision-making structure.

62 In broad terms Sigurd Bu in 1941 held that state hospitals generally to a much greater extent than local authority or private hospitals were open for patients from all of Norway. Bu, *Sykehusene*, 5. Extensive research, however, is necessary to qualify this statement.

63 Bu, *Sykehusene*, 88.

Conclusion

Let us suggest some very preliminary conclusions. Evidence, mainly based on mid 1930s reports from local and regional authorities and district and county medical officers, suggests, somewhat unexpectedly, that access to hospitals for rural and remote populations was quite satisfactory, excepting the 'periphery of the periphery', where communications were especially problematic. Inhabitants of rural or peripheral areas were admitted to both local authority and private hospitals, most often located in urban areas, in much the same way and on the same conditions as town-dwellers. City or town hospitals were often planned to cater also for their respective rural environs, whose government and other agencies often took part in planning and made financial contributions. All this reflected very strong localist approaches, with the resulting highly decentralised structure characteristic of Norwegian hospital building. Similarly national tendencies towards local authority welfare or tripartite cooperation between local authorities, the state and private humanitarian welfare organisations were influential. How was this possible in a not too prosperous country under difficult economic circumstances in the 1920s and 30s? One answer is that most hospitals at the time were low-tech and low-cost institutions. They had only one or a few doctors, and nursing was often more of a mission than an occupation, featuring low pay for long hours. Many hospitals relied heavily upon voluntary and spare time assistance, both for administration and physical construction and maintenance. Food could be purchased directly from local farmers and supporters collected money from lotteries and sponsors, sewed bed-linen, made furniture, or picked wild berries for the hospital's supply of jam.[64]

Hospital treatment costs were a problem for many though; more so for rural and peripheral populations than for urban dwellers, essentially because of the lower ratio of rural wage-earners. Until the health insurance scheme was extended from the mid-1930s, rural and peripheral dwellers were more likely to be excluded and required to pay from their own purses or to ask for social support that did not come easy and was often considered socially stigmatising. Patients from the countryside also were likely to face charges for extras and that part of day-rates that health insurance did not cover. Such problems would have been still greater had the hospitals made patients or their respective home authorities pay the full real costs. Instead, at least in some cases, deficits were covered by tax-moneys from the inhabitants of the host community, more often than not urban people. Later the problem of hospital expenses for patients, whether rural or urban, all but disappeared with the universal health benefits of the mid-late 1950s.

---

64 Reiersen, *Sykehuset Sanitetsforeningen Lokalsamfunnet*; Jacobsen, *Fra sneppert til skalpell*.

Quality, as measured by the degree of specialisation, was low, and this was the case nationwide, excepting the capital Oslo and very few other cities. Around half of the 20 counties were affected by an especially low degree of specialisation, with no or extremely few specialists outside of surgery. Also, there was no formal hierarchy or regionalisation, and though the National Hospital was, in principle, open to all, access seems to have been quite restricted. We know little of other informal hierarchies, although Bergen apparently functioned quite well as a centre of specialisation for much of West Norway.

It could be argued, then, that the highly decentralised, locally initiated structure, and the resulting relatively good access to hospitals for rural and peripheral areas of Norway, came at the price of a low degree of specialisation in hospitals, and an equally low degree of formal hierarchies. These problems were exacerbated after World War Two with rapidly growing demand for high quality hospital treatments; a steadily growing intolerance of inequality; and simultaneously increasing perceptions as to the meanings and practical expressions of equality. The strong localist ties of Norwegian hospitals have, however, continued to be highly viable. Thus, the tension between securing easy and equal access to hospitals in a geographically wide, subdivided and sparsely populated country, and on the other hand improving quality of care through a high degree of specialisation and concentration, has been marked in Norway, imprinting heavily on Norwegian hospital policies and conflicts to this day.[65]

65 Grønlie, 'Norwegian General Hospitals'.

SELECT BIBLIOGRAPHY

This is a brief guide to accessible literature relevant to health issues in rural Europe during the period. In addition to the areas covered by chapters in this volume (see also relevant footnotes), brief sections on Germany and Russia are included.

EUROPEAN AND INTERNATIONAL

Baldwin, P. *Contagion and the State in Europe 1830-1930*, Cambridge, Cambridge University Press, 1999.

Barnes, D.S. *The Great Stink of Paris and the Nineteenth Century Struggle against Filth and Germs*, Baltimore, Johns Hopkins University Press, 2006.

Barona, J.L. 'Nutrition and Health. The International Context during the Inter-war Crisis', *Social History of Medicine*, 21, (2008), 87-105.

Barona, J.L. and Cherry, S. (eds.) *Health and Medicine in Rural Europe 1850-1945,* València, PUV, Seminari d'Estudis sobre la Ciència, 2005.

Blecourt, W. and Usbourne, C. (eds.) *Cultural Approaches to the History of Medicine. Mediating Medicine in Early Modern and Modern Europe*, Basingstoke, Palgrave, 2004.

Borowy, I. and Gruner, W.D. (eds.) *Facing Illness in Troubled Times*, Frankfurt am Main, Peter Lang, 2005.

Brunton, D. (ed.) *Medicine Transformed: Health, Disease and Society in Europe 1800-1930,* Manchester, Manchester University/Open University Press, 2004.

Bynum, W.F; Hardy, A; Jacyna, S; Lawrence, C; Tansey, E.M. *The Western Medical Tradition 1800 to 2000,* Cambridge, Cambridge University Press, 2000.

Bynum, W.F. *Science and the Practice of Medicine in the Nineteenth Century*, Cambridge, Cambridge University Press, 1994.

Cherry, S. (ed.) 'Medicine and rural health care in 19th and early 20th century Europe'. Special Issue, *Journal of Regional and Local Studies*, 2, (2006).

Freeman, R. *The Politics of Health in Europe*, Manchester, Manchester University Press, 2000.

Harrison, M. *Disease and the Modern World*, Cambridge, Polity Press, 2004.

Huisman. F. and Warner, J.H. (eds.) *Locating Medical History. The Stories and their Meanings*, Baltimore, Johns Hopkins University Press, 2004.

Imhof, A.E. *Lost Worlds. How Our European Ancestors Coped With Everyday Life and Why Life is so Hard Today*, Charlottesville, University of Virginia Press, 1996.

Jutte, R; Ecklof, M; and Nelson, M. (eds.) *Historical Aspects of Unconventional Medicine,* Sheffield, European Association for the History of Medicine and Health, 2001.

McKeown, T. *The Modern Rise of Population,* London, Edward Arnold, 1976.

Milward, A. and Saul, S. B. *The Development of the Economies of Continental Europe,* London, Allen and Unwin, 1977.

Mitchell, B.R. *International Historical Statistics: Europe 1750-1988,* Basingstoke, Macmillan, 1992.

Phillips, H. and Killingray, D. (eds.) *The Spanish Influenza Pandemic of 1918-19,* London, Routledge, 2003.

Pickstone, J. *Ways of Knowing: A New History of Science, Technology and Medicine*, Manchester, Manchester University Press, 2000.

Porter, D. (ed.) *The History of Public Health and the Modern State*, Amsterdam, Rodopi, 1994.
Porter, R. *The Greatest Benefit to Mankind*, London, Harper Collins, 1997.
Porter, R. (ed.) *The Popularisation of Medicine 1650-1850*, London, Routledge, 1992.
Pratt, A.C. 'Discourses of Rurality: Loose Talk or Social Struggle', *Journal of Rural Studies,* 12, (1996), 69-78.
Schofield, R; Rehrer, D.; Bideau, A. *The Decline of Mortality in Europe,* Oxford, Clarendon Press, 1991.
Voegele, J. and Woelk, W. (eds.) *Stadt, Krankenheit und Tod wahrend der Epidemiologischen Transition*, Berlin, Duncker & Humblot, 2000.
Weindling, P. 'Health and Medicine in Interwar Europe'. In Cooter, R. and Pickstone, J. (eds.) *Companion to Medicine in the Twentieth Century*, Amsterdam, Harwood Academic, 2003, 29-50.
Weindling, P. *Epidemics and Genocide in Eastern Europe 1890-1945*, Cambridge, Cambridge University Press, 1995.

BRITAIN

Abel Smith, B. *The Hospitals*, London, Heinemann, 1964.
Armstrong, A. *The Population of Victorian and Edwardian Norfolk,* Norwich, Centre of East Anglian Studies, UEA, 2000.
Berridge, V. *Opium and the People. Opiate Use and Drug Control Policy in Nineteenth and early Twentieth Century England,* London, Free Association Books, 1999.
Bynum, W. F. Lock, S.; Porter, R. *Medical Journals and Medical Knowledge*, London, Routledge, 1992, 228-247.
Cherry, S. 'Medicine and Public Health 1900-39'. In Wrigley, C. (ed.) *Companion to Early Twentieth Century Britain,* Oxford, Blackwell, 2004, 405-423.
Cherry, S. *Medical Services and the Hospitals in Britain, 1860-1939,* Cambridge, Cambridge University Press, 1996.
Cherry, S. 'Change and continuity in cottage hospitals 1859-1948', *Medical History*, 36, (1992), 271-89.
Cooter, R. (ed.) *In the Name of the Child: Health and Welfare 1880-1940*, London, Routledge, 1992.
Cooter, R. (ed.) *Studies in the history of alternative medicine*, London, Macmillan, 1988.
Crowther, M.A. *The Workhouse System 1834-1929*, London, Methuen, 1981.
Davies, C. 'The health visitor as mother's friend', *Social History of Medicine, 5,* (1993), 39-60.
Davin, A. 'Imperialism and Motherhood', *History Workshop*, *5*, (1978), 9-65.
Digby, A. and Bosanquet, N. 'Doctors and patients in an era of national health insurance and private practice, 1913-38', *Economic History Review*, XLI, (1988), 74-94.
Digby, A. *The Evolution of British General Practice 1850-1948*, Oxford, Clarendon Press, 1999.
Digby, A. *Making a Medical Living*, Cambridge, Cambridge University Press, 1994.
Donnison, J. *Midwives and Medical Men*, New Barnet, Historical Publications, 1988.
Dyehouse, C. 'Working Class Mothers and Infant Mortality in England 1895-1918', *Journal of Social History, 12* (1978), 248-67.
Emrys Roberts, M. *The Cottage Hospitals 1859-1990*, Motcombe, Tern, 1991.
Fee, E. and Porter, D. 'Public health, preventive medicine and professionalisation', in Wear, A. (ed.) *Medicine in Society,* 265-275.

Granshaw, L. 'Fame and fortune by means of bricks and mortar'. In Granshaw, L. and Porter, R. (eds.), *The Hospital in History*, London, Routledge, 1989, 199-220.
Hamilton, C. 'Sanitary policing and the local state', *Social History of Medicine, 18*, (2005), 39-61.
Hamlin, C. *Public Health and Social Justice in the Age of Chadwick: Britain 1800-1854*, Cambridge, Cambridge University Press, 1998.
Hamlin, C. 'State Medicine in Great Britain' in Porter, R. *The History of Public Health and the Modern State*, 132-164.
Hardy, A. *Health and Medicine in Britain since 1860*, Basingstoke, Palgrave, 2001.
Hardy, A. *The Epidemic Streets*, Oxford, Clarendon Press, 1993.
Hirst, J.D. 'The growth of treatment through the School Medical Service 1908-18', *Social History of Medicine, 1,* (1988), 318-42.
Lawrence, C. *Medicine in the Making of Modern Britain, 1700-1920,* London, Routledge, 1994.
Loudon, I. (ed.) *Western Medicine: An Illustrated History*, Oxford, Oxford University Press, 1997.
Loudon, I. 'On Maternal and Infant Mortality 1900-60', *Social History of Medicine, 4*, (1991) 29-73.
Loudon, I. and Drury, M. 'Some aspects of clinical care in General Practice'. In Loudon, I.; Webster, C.; Horder, J. (eds.) *General Practice under the National Health Service 1948-97*, Oxford, Clarendon Press, 1997, 92-127.
Palmengiano, E.M. *Health and British Magazines in the Nineteenth Century*, Lanham, Scarecrow Press, 1998.
Porter, R. *Disease, Medicine and Society in England, 1550-1860*, Cambridge, Cambridge University Press, 1993.
Ranger, T. and Slack, P. (eds.) *Epidemics and Ideas,* Cambridge, Cambridge University Press, 1992.
Riley, J.C. *Sick, not Dead*, Baltimore, Johns Hopkins University Press, 1997.
Riley, J.C. *The Eighteenth Century Campaign to Avoid Disease*, Basingstoke, Macmillan, 1987.
Saks, M. *Alternative Medicine*, Oxford, Clarendon Press, 1992.
Smith, F.B. *The People's Health 1830-1910*, London, Wiedenfeld and Nicolson, 1979.
Sturdy, S. (ed.) *Medicine, Health and the Public Sphere in Britain 1600-2000,* London, Routledge, 2002.
Szreter, S. 'The importance of social intervention in Britain's nineteenth century mortality decline', *Social History of Medicine, 1*, (1988), 1-18.
Waller, P.J. *Town, City and Nation: England 1870-1914*, Oxford, Oxford University Press, 1983.
Wear, A. (ed.) *Medicine in Society,* Cambridge, Cambridge University Press, 1992.
Webster, C. (ed.) *Caring for Health: history and diversity*, Buckingham, Open University Press, 1993.
Weindling, P. 'From infectious to chronic diseases: changing patterns of sickness in the 19th and 20th centuries' in Wear, A. (ed.) *Medicine in Society*, 303-316.
Williams, R. *The Country and the City*, London, The Hogarth Press, 1973.
Wohl, A. *Endangered Lives: Public Health in Victorian Britain*, London, Dent, 1983.
Worboys, M. *Spreading Germs: disease theories and medical practice in Britain 1865-1900,* Cambridge, Cambridge University Press, 2002

FRANCE

Ackerman, E.B. *Health Care in the Parisian Countryside 1800-1914*, New Brunswick, Rutgers University Press, 1997.

Barnes, D.S. *The Making of a Social Disease: Tuberculosis in Nineteenth Century France*, Berkeley, University of California Press, 1995.

Bourdelais, P. (ed.) *Les hygienists; Enjeux, modeles et practiques (XVIIIe-Xxe siecles)*, Paris, Belin, 2000.

Bourdelais, P; Faure, O. *Les nouvelles pratiques de santé. XVIII-XXe siècles*, Paris, Belin, 2005.

Dinges, M. 'Social History of Medicine in Germany and France in the late Twentieth Century'. In Huisman and Warner, *Locating Medical History*, 209-36.

Châtelet, A-M. *L'école de plein air. Une expérience pédagogique et architecturale dans l'Europe du XXe siècle*, Focales, Editions Recherches, 2003.

De Luca, V. *Aux origines de l'Etat-Providence. Les inspecteurs de l'Assistance publique et l'aide sociale à l'enfance (1820-1930)*, Paris, Ined, 2002.

Faure, O. *Les Français et leur medicine*, Paris, Belin, 1993.

Faure, O. 'The Social History of Health in France: a survey of recent developments', *Social History of Medicine, 3,* (1990), 437-451.

La Berge, A.F. 'The early 19th century French Public Health Movement', *Bulletin History of Medicine*, 58, (1984), 3, 363-379.

McPhee, P. *A Social History of France,* London, Routledge, 1992.

Norvez, A. *De la naissance à l'école. Santé, modes de garde et préscolarité dans la France contemporaine*, Paris, Ined/Puf, 1990.

Ramsey, M. 'The popularisation of medicine in France, 1650-1890'. In Porter, *Popularisation of Medical Knowledge*, 97-133.

Renouard, J-M. *De l'enfant coupable à l'enfant abandonné. Le traitement scial et politique de la deviance*, Païdos, Histoire, Centurion, 1990.

Rollet, C. *Les carnets de santé des enfants,* Paris, La Dispute, 2008.

Rollet, C. *Les enfants au XIXe siècle*, Paris, Hachette, 2001.

Rollet, C. *La politique à l'égard de la petite enfance sous la Troisième République*, Paris, PUF/Ined, 1990.

Spears, J. 'Folk medicine and popular attitudes towards disease in the High Alps 1780-1870', *Bulletin History of Medicine*, 54, (1980), 3, 303-336.

Weber, E. *La fin des terroirs. La modernisation de la France rurale 1870-1914*, Paris, Fayard, 1983.

GERMANY

Berg, M. and Cocks, G. (eds.) *Medicine and Modernity. Public health and medical care in 19th and 20th century Germany*, Cambridge, Cambridge University Press, 1997.

Bleker, J. 'To benefit the poor and advance medical science. Hospitals and hospital care in Germany 1820-1870'. In Berg and Cocks, *Medicine and Modernity,* 17-34.

Evans, R. *Death in Hamburg. Society and Politics in the Cholera Years*, Harmondsworth, Penguin, 1990.

Faltin, T. *Heil und Heilung. Geschichte der Laienheilkundigen und Struktur anti-modernisitscher Weltanschauungen in Kaiserreich und Weimarer Republik*, Stuttgart, Franz Steiner, 2000.

Fassl, P. and Kiessling, R. (eds.) *Volksleben im 19 Jahrhundert. Studien zu den bayerischen Physikatsberichten und verwandten Quellen*, Augsburg, Wissner, 2003.

Gockenjan, G. *Kurieren und Staat machen. Gesundheit und Medizin in der burgerlichen Welt*, Frankfurt, Suhrkamp, 1985

Heller, R. 'Priest Doctors as a rural health service in the age of Enlightenment', *Medical History, 20*, (1976), 361-83.

Heller, R. 'Johan Christian Reil's training scheme for medical auxiliaries', *Medical History 19*, (1975), 321-332.

Heuerkamp, C. *Der Aufstieg der Artze im 19.Jahrhundert*, Göttingen, Vandenhoeck & Ruprecht, 1985.

Labisch, A. 'From traditional individualism to collective professionalism'. In Berg and Cocks, *Medicine and Modernity,* 35-54.

Labisch, A. *Homo Hygienicus. Gesundheit und Medizin in der Neuzeit*, Frankfurt, Campus, 1992.

Molitor, J. 'Zwei Physikatsberichte des Landgerichtes Deggendorf aus den Jahren 1830 und 1860', *Deggendorfer Gesichtsblatter*, 6, (1986), 99-143.

Raeff, M. *The well-ordered police state...the Germanies and Russia*, New Haven, Yale University Press, 1983.

Ross, C. *Naked Germany. Health, Race and the Nation*, Hamburg, Berg, 2005.

Schenda, R. 'Stadtmedizin – Landmedizin. Ein Versuch zur Eklarung subkulturellen medikalen Verhaltens'. In Kaufmann, G. (ed.) *Stadt-Land Beziehungen*, Göttingen, Schwartz, 1975, 147-169.

Spree, R. *Health and Social Class in Imperial Germany*, Hamburg, Berg, 1988.

Stolberg, M. 'National statistics on the causes of death in nineteenth-century Bavaria', *Journal of the History of Medicine and Allied Services*, 54, (1999), 210-255.

Stolberg, M. 'Patientenschaft und Krankheitspectrum im landlichen Artzpraxen des 19. Jahrhunderts', *Medizinhistorisches Journal*, 28, (1993), 3-27.

Stolberg, M. 'Alternative Medicine, irregular healers and the medical market in Bavaria'. In Jutte, Eklof and Nelson, *Historical Aspects of Unconventional Medicine*, 139-161.

Tuchman, A.M. 'The true assistant to the obstetrician': State regulation and the legal protection of midwives in 19th century Prussia', *Social History of Medicine*, *18*, (2005), 1, 23-38.

Voegele, J. *Urban Mortality Change in England and Germany, 1870-1913*, Liverpool, Liverpool University Press, 1998.

Weindling, P. 'Medicine and Modernisation: the social history of German health and medicine', *History of Science*, *24*, (1986), 277-301.

ITALY

Berlinguer, G. *Storia e politica della salute*, Milan, Angeli, 1991.

Betri, M.L. and Gigli Marchetti, A. (eds.) *Salute e classi lavoratrici in Italia dall'Unità al Fascismo,* Milan, Angeli, 1982.

Breschi, M. and Pozzi, L. (eds.) *Salute, Malattia e Sopravvivenza in Italia 1800 e 1900*, Udine, Forum, 2007.

Bussini, O. and Lanari, D. 'Statura e condizioni di salute della popolazione maschile a fine Ottocento: uno studio basato sui registri di leva'. In Breschi and Pozzi (eds.) *Salute, Malattia e Sopravvivenza in Italia,* 105-33

Caselli, G. 'Mortalità e sopravvivenza in Italia dall'Unità agli anni '30.' In *Popolazione, Società e Ambiente*, Bologna, CLUEB, 1987

Cau, P.; Merella, C.; Pozzi, L. 'Lo stato di salute della popolazione di Alghero fra 1800 e 1900. Uno studio condotto attraverso i registri militari.' In Breschi and Pozzi, *Salute, Malattia e Sopravvivenza in Italia*, 135-56.

Corsini, C.A. (ed.) *Statura, salute e migrazioni: le leve militari italiane*, Udine, Forum, 2008.

Cosmacini, G. *Storia della Medicina e della Sanità in Italia. Dalla peste nera ai nostri giorni*, Bari-Roma, Laterza, 2005.

De Bernardi, A. *Il mal della rosa. Denutrizione e pellagra nelle campagne italiane fra 1800 e 1900*, Milano, Angeli, 1984.

Delogu, S. *Storia di una Malattia Sociale: il Tracoma in Sardegna dal 1900 al 1950.* Tesi di Laurea. Facoltà di Giurisprudenza, Corso di Laurea in *Scienze Politiche* (Relatore Prof. F. Manconi), Università degli Studi di Sassari, 1990-1991.

Della Peruta, F. (ed.) *Storia d'Italia, Annali VII, Malattia e Medicina*, Torino, Einaudi, 1984.

Gatti, A.M. and Puggioni, G. 'Storia della popolazione dal 1847 a oggi.' In Berlinguer, L. and Mattone, A. (eds.) *La Sardegna*, Torino, G. Einaudi, 1998.

Gatti, A.M.; Calò, C.M.; Piras, I.S. 'Lo stato di salute delle leve militari in Sardegna tra Ottocento e Novecento'. In Corsini, C.A. (ed.) *Statura, salute e migrazioni,* 169-91.

Le Lannou, M. *Pastori e contadini di Sardegna*, IV Italian Edition (M. Brigaglia transl. of *Pâtres et paysans de la Sardaigne*, Tours, Arrault, 1941). Cagliari, Edizioni Della Torre, 2006.

Luzzo, S. *Salute e sanità nell'Italia repubblicana*, Rome, Donzelli, 2004.

Mann, I. *Culture, Race, Climate and Eye Disease*, Springfield Illinois, Charles C. Thomas, 1966.

Newell Hofmann, E. *Sources of Mortality Changes in Italy since Unification*, New York, Arno Press, 1981.

Pozzi, L. *La lotta per la vita. Evoluzione e geografia della sopravvivenza in Italia* fra 1800 e 1900, Udine, Forum, 2000.

Pozzi, L. and Tognotti L. (eds.) 'Salute e malattia fra 1800 e 1900' in *Sardegna e nei paesi dell'Europa mediterranea,* Edes, Sassari, 2000.

Sormani, G. 'Geografia nosologica d'Italia', in Dirstat MAIC *Annali di Statistica*, serie II, vol. VI. 1881.

Taylor, H. *Trachoma: A Blinding Scourge from the Bronze Age to the Twenty First Century,* East Melbourne Victoria Centre for Eye Research, Haddington Press, 2008.

Tognotti, E. *La malaria in Sardegna. Per una storia del paludismo nel Mezzogiorno 1880-1950*, Milan, Angeli, 1996.

NORWAY

Andresen, A. 'A farewell to "Rural Bliss". Shifting problematizations of school children's health in Norway 1900 – 1940', *Scandinavian Journal of History*, 33 (3), 2008, 169-288.

Andresen, A. and Ryymin, T. 'Rural Health and the Norwegian Health Acts of 1860 and 1912'. In Barona, J.L. and Cherry, S. (eds.) *Health and Medicine in Rural Europe 1850-1945*, València, PUV, Seminari d'Estudis sobre la Ciència, 2005.

Bjørnson, Ø.; Haavet, I. E. *Langsomt ble landet et velferdssamfunn. Trygdens historie 1894-1994*, Oslo, AdNotam Gyldendal, 1994.

Elstad, I. and Hamran, T. *Sykdom. Nord-Norge før 1940*, Bergen, Fagbokforlaget, 2006.

Grønlie, T. 'Velferdskommune og utjevningststat'. In Næss, H.E. et al. *Folkestyre i by og bygd*, Oslo, Bergen, Stavanger, Tromsø, Universitetsforlaget, 1987.

Hubbard, W. et al. *Historical Studies in Mortality Decline*, Det Norske Videnskaps-Akademi, Oslo, 2002.

Larsen, Ø. (ed.) *The Shaping of a Profession. Physicians in Norway, Past and Present*, Canton, Mass., Science History Publications, 1996.

Nagel, A.-H. (ed.) *Velferdskommunen. Kommunenes rolle i utviklingen av velferdsstaten*, Bergen, Alma Mater, 1991.

Ryymin, T. *Smitte, språk og kultur. Tuberkulosearbeidet i Finnmark 1900 – 1960*, Oslo, Scandinavian Academic Press/Spartacus, 2009.

Ryymin, T. and Andresen, A. 'Effecting Equality. Norwegian Health Policy in Finnmark 1845 – 1970s', *Acta Borealia*, 2009, 26:1, 96 – 114.

Schiøtz, A. *Det offentlige helsevesen i Norge 1603-2003. Folkets helse –landets styrke 1850 – 2003*, Oslo, Universitetsforlaget, 2003.

Schiøtz, A. *Doktoren. Distriktslegenes historie 1900 – 1984*, Oslo, Pax Forlag A/S, 2003.

Seip, A.L. *Veiene til velferdsstaten. Norsk sosialpolitikk 1920 – 75,* Oslo, Gyldendal, 1994.

RUSSIA

Cherry, S. 'Medicine and the Russian peasantry: revisiting zemstvo health care c. 1864-1917'. In Andresen, A; Grønlie, T.; Ryymin, T. (eds.) *Science, Culture, Politics. European Perspectives on Medicine, Sickness and Health*, Bergen, Stein Rokkan Centre for Social Studies, 4, 2006, 155-172.

Frieden, N. *Russian Physicians in an era of Reform and Revolution 1856-1905*, New Jersey, Princeton University Press, 1981.

Frieden, N. 'Child care: medical reform in a traditionalist culture'. In Ransel, D.L. (ed.) *The Family in Imperial Russia,* 220-45.

Glickman, R.L. 'The Peasant Woman as Healer'. In Clements, E.B; Engel, E.A; and Worobec, C.W. *Russia's Women*, Berkeley, University of California Press, 1991 vol.1, 148-62.

Haines, A. J. *Health Work in Soviet Russia*, New York, Vanguard Press, 1928.

Hutchinson, J.F. 'Who killed Cock Robin? - an enquiry into the death of Zemstvo medicine'. In Solomon and Hutchinson, *Health and Society in Revolutionary Russia*, 1-15.

Krug, P.F. 'The debate over the delivery of health care in rural Russia: the Moscow Zemstvo, 1864-1878,' *Bulletin History of Medicine*, *50*, (1976), 2, 226-41.

Pratt, J.K. 'The Free Economic Society and the battle against smallpox', *The Russian Review*, *61*, (2002), 560-78.

Ramer, S.C. 'The zemstvo and public health'. In Emmons, T and Vucinich, W.S. *The Zemstvo in Russia: An experiment in local self-government*, Cambridge, Cambridge University Press, 1982, 279-314.

Ransel, D.L. *Village Mothers: Three generations of change in Russia and Tataria*, Bloomington, Indiana University Press, 2003.

Ransel, D.L. (ed.) *The Family in Imperial Russia,* Chicago, University of Illinois Press, 1978.

Ryan, M. *The Organisation of Soviet Medical Care*, Oxford, Blackwell, 1998.

Sigerist, H. *Medicine and Health in the Soviet Union*, New York, Citadel Press, 1947.

Soloman, S.G. and Hutchinson, J.F (eds.) *Health and Society in Revolutionary Russia*, Bloomington, Indiana University Press, 1990.

Tian-Shanskaia, O. *Village Life in Tsarist Russia* (transl. Ransel, D.), Bloomington, Indiana University Press, Bloomington, 1993.

SPAIN

Atenza Fernández, J. and Martínez Pérez, J. (eds.) *El centro secundario de higiene rural de Talavera de la Reina y la sanidad española de su tiempo*, Toledo, Junta de Castilla La Mancha, 2001.

Báguena Cervellera, M.J. 'Saberes y prácticas en torno a la polio en la medicina valenciana 1900-1950'. In Martínez Pérez, J.; Porras Gallo, M.I.; Del Cura González, M. (eds.) *La Medicina en el nuevo milenio. Una perspectiva historica*, Cuenca, Ed. UCLM, 2004, 949-962.

Barona Vilar, C. *Las políticas de la salud,* Valencia, PUV, 2005.

Barona, J.L. 'Health, medicine and cultural interaction in rural Spain 1875-1936', *International Journal of Regional and Local Studies*, series 2, (2006), 31-51.

Barona, J.L.'The European Conference of Rural health and the Spanish Administration'. In Barona, J.L. and Cherry, S. (eds.) *Health and Medicine in Rural Europe 1850-1945,* Valencia, SEC-PUV, 2005, 127-146.

Barona, J.L. 'Condicions de vida a l'horta valenciana. El testimoni dels metges', *Afers*, 19, (2004), 67-92.

Barona, J.L. *Salud, enfermedad y muerte. La sociedad valenciana entre 1833 y 1939*, València, Institució Alfons el Magnànim, 2003.

Barona, J.L; Bernabeu-Mestre, J; Perdiguero, E. 'Health Problems and Public Policies in Rural Spain'. In Barona, J.L. and Cherry, S. (eds.) *Health and Medicine in Rural Europe 1850-1941*, València, Seminari d'Estudis sobre la Ciència, 2005, 63-82.

Barona, J.L. and Bernabeu, J. *La salud y el estado. El movimiento sanitario internacional y la administración'*, in Barona, J.L. and Cherry, S. (eds.) *Health and Medicine in Rural Europe 1850-1941*, Valencia, SEC, 2003; 287-303.

Bernabeu-Mestre, J. *La salut pública que no va poder ser. José Estellés Salarich 1896-1990: una aportació valenciana a la sanitat espanyola contemporània*, València, Consell Valencià de Cultura, 2007.

Bernabeu-Mestre, J. 'State of Health of the Catalan Areas: the Work of the Acadèmia d'Higiene', in Barona, J.L.; Cortell, E.; Perdiguero, E. (eds.) *Medi ambient i salut en els municipis valencians. Una perspectiva històrica*, Sueca, Seminari d'Estudis sobre la Ciencia/Ajuntament de Sueca, 2002.

Bernabeu-Mestre, J; Galiana, M.E; Esplugues, J.X. and Cid, P. 'Overexploitation, malnutrition and stigma in a women's illness: chlorosis in contemporary Spanish medicine 1877-1936', in Harris, B; Gálvez, L; Machado, E. (eds.) *Gender and wellbeing in Europe: historical and contemporary perspectives*, Hampshire: Ashgate, 2009, 154-171.

Bernabeu-Mestre, J.; Esplugues, J.X.; Pascual, M.; Terol. V, (eds) *Salut i societat en els municipis valencians: una perspectiva histórica*, Valencia. Denes, 2008.

Bernabeu-Mestre, J.; Perdiguero, E.; Barona, J. L. 'Determinanti della mortalità infantile e transizione sanitaria. Una riflesione a partire dall'esperienza spagnola'. In Breschi, M.; Pozzi, L. (eds.) *Salute, malattia e sopravivenza in Italia fra 1800 e 1900*, Udine, Forum, 2007; 175-193.

Bernabeu-Mestre, J.; Caballero, P.; Nolasco, A.; Galiana. M.E. 'Niveles de vida y salud en la España del primer franquismo: las desigualdades en la mortalidad infantil', *Revista de Demografía Histórica*, 24, 2006, 173-193.

Bernabeu-Mestre, J.; Robles, E.; Esplugues, J.X. (eds.) *Higiene y salubritat en els municipis valencians 1813-1939*, Benissa, Seminari d'Estudis sobre la Ciencia/Institut d'Estudis Comarcals de la Marina Alta, 1997.

Galiana-Sánchez, ME; Bernabeu-Mestre, J. 'El problema sanitario de España: saneamiento y medio rural en los primeros decenios del siglo XX', *Asclepio*, 58 (2006), 139-164.

Guillem-Llobat, X. 'El paper dels laboratoris municipals valencians en el control de qualitat dels aliments 1881-1936', *Actes D'Història de la Ciència i de la Tècnica* 1 (2008), 293-300.

Guillem-Llobat, X. *El control de la qualitat dels aliments. El cas valencià en el context internacional 1878-1936*, Valencia, PUV, 2007.

Jiménez Lucena, I. 'La Segunda República, una apuesta por la higiene rural: el nivel legislativo.' In *Actas del XXXIII Congreso Internacional de Historia de la Medicina. Granada-Sevilla, 1-6 Septiembre 1992*. Sevilla, 1994, 567-580.

Martínez Carrión, J.M. (ed.) *El nivel de vida en la España rural, siglos XVIII-XX*, Alicante, Universidad de Alicante, 2002.

Perdiguero Gil, E. (comp.) *Salvad al niño. Estudios sobre la protección a la infancia en la Europa mediterránea a comienzos del siglo XX*, Valencia, PUV/SEC, 2004.

Perdiguero Gil, E.; Castejón, R. (eds.) 'La acción social de la medicina y la construcción del sistema sanitario contemporáneo en España', *Trabajo Social y Salud (Monográfico)*, 43, 2002.

Rodríguez Ocaña, E. 'La Salud pública en la España de la primera mitad del siglo XX'. In Atenza, J.; Martínez, J. (eds.) *El Centro Secundario de Higiene rural de Talavera de la Reina y la sanidad española de su tiempo*. Toledo, JCCM, 2001, 37- 48.

Rodríguez Ocaña, E. 'The politics of Public Health in the State-Managed Scheme of Healthcare in Spain 1940-1990'. In Löwy, I.; Krige, J. (eds.) *Images of Disease. Science, Public Policy and Health in Post-war Europe*, Luxembourg, European Communities Pub., 2001, 187-210.

Rodríguez Ocaña, E. and Martínez Navarro, F. *Salud pública en España. De la Edad Media al siglo XXI*, Granada, Escuela Andaluza de Salud Pública, 2009.

Rodríguez-Ocaña, E. and Menéndez-Navarro, A. 'La tardía intervención higiénica en el medio rural español: el caso de la lucha contra la anquilostomiasis, 1910-1960'. *La Mutua*, 2ª época, n. 16, 2006, 71-86.

Rodríguez Ocaña, E. and Perdiguero, E. (eds.) 'Ciencia y persuasión social en la medicalización de la infancia en España, siglos XIX-XX', *História, Ciências, Saúde Manguinhos (Monográfico)*, 13 (2006).

Salort Vives, S. *Vivir y morir en Alicante. Higienistas e inversiones públicas en salud 1859-1923*, Alicante, Publicaciones Universidad de Alicante, 2008.

www.ingramcontent.com/pod-product-compliance
Ingram Content Group UK Ltd.
Pitfield, Milton Keynes, MK11 3LW, UK
UKHW021832100926
8556IPUK00004B/301

9 783631 596531